STRAIGHT TALK

TALK

about

BREAST CANCER

FROM DIAGNOSIS TO RECOVERY

Fifth Edition

Suzanne W. Braddock, M.D.

Jane M. Kercher, M.D.

John J. Edney, M.D.

Margaret Block, M.D.

Melanie Morrissey Clark

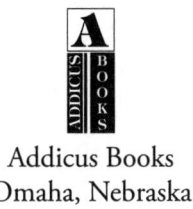

Addicus Books

Omaha, Nebraska

An Addicus Nonfiction Book

ISBN: 978-1-940495-70-5
Cover design by Peri Poloni-Gabriel
Typography and illustrations by Jack Kusler

This book is not intended to serve as a substitute for a physician. Nor is it the authors' intent to give medical advice contrary to that of an attending physician.

All proceeds from the sale of this book are donated to the *Straight Talk about Breast Cancer Charitable Trust* and are used to assist breast cancer patients and their families.

Library of Congress Cataloging-in-Publication Data

Braddock, Suzanne W., 1942-
  Straight talk about breast cancer : from diagnosis to recovery / Suzanne W. Braddock [and four others]. — Fifth edition.
      pages cm
  Previous ed.: Straight talk about breast cancer / Suzanne W. Braddock ... [et al.]. 2010.
  Includes bibliographical references and index.
  ISBN 978-1-940495-70-5 (paperback)
  1. Breast—Cancer—Popular works. I. Title.
  RC280.B8S748 2015
  616.99'449—dc23

                                                    2014033745

Addicus Books, Inc.
P.O. Box 45327
Omaha, Nebraska 68145
www.AddicusBooks.com

Printed in the United States of America
10 9 8 7 6 5 4 3 2 1

*To all the women with breast cancer,
their families, and their loved ones*

Contents

Preface

$\mathcal{P}$lease read this book imagining that a very good friend is sitting close to you, giving you this introduction to the rest of your life with love and understanding. Imagine your friend—who has indeed walked in your shoes—taking you by the hand and guiding you through the next few weeks.

Your friend wants to help you understand what is happening, and help you cope with the decisions and treatments ahead. She also wants to help your family and friends, for they are suffering with you.

Know there will come a time when you'll go entire minutes without thinking of breast cancer—then hours, and even days. Of course, your life will never be the same. In fact, it will probably be better in many ways you would not have chosen but will be delighted to discover.

The authors of this book reach out to you as dear friends and offer you the hope of a complete recovery, along with the certainty that the journey from here will be one of growth, challenge, and change. That is, after all, what life is about.

Acknowledgments

We, the authors, would like to thank those who helped make this book possible. We are grateful to physicians Robert Langdon Jr., M.D., Patrick McKenna, M.D., Janalyn Prows, M.D., Henry Lynch, M.D., Ramon Fusaro, M.D., John J. Heieck, M.D., Richard Bruneteau, M.D., and Carol Kornhehl, M.D., author of *The Best News about Radiation Therapy.*

We thank Mollie Foster, Ph.D., for her contributions and Judy Dierkhising, Ph.D., for her insights into the emotional needs of breast cancer patients. Our appreciation goes to the Nebraska Methodist Hospital Breast Cancer Support Group for their comments, wit, and strength. And with gratitude, we remember Sue Kocsis, a real spark, whose encouragement meant so much during the early stages of this book.

We are also deeply grateful to the women who shared their personal stories in order to help others. A special thanks to the women who shared their surgery and reconstruction photos. We acknowledge photographers Larry Ferguson and Paula Friedland for their creativity and sensitivity in portraying these women as real, living people, rather than medical subjects. We thank Jack Kusler, who provided illustrations and designed the layout of the book.

Introduction

ſomeone you love or someone you know will get breast cancer—your friend, your aunt, your mother, your father, your daughter, yourself. The fact is, if you are an American woman, your chance of getting breast cancer is especially high—about one in eight over your lifetime. The chance of dying from breast cancer is one in thirty-six. Each year in the United States, more than 200,000 women are diagnosed with breast cancer.

Here's the good news: Thanks to early detection and better ways to treat breast cancer, more and more women with breast cancer are surviving. The percentage has climbed steadily since 1989—not just five-year disease-free survival, either, but real, lasting, bounce-the-grandkids-on-your-knee survival.

The rest of my life started April 1, 1992, with a phone call from my friend and doctor, who informed me that the lump in my breast was malignant. I reacted, as do most women, with the irrational certainty that I was going to die, and soon. I was forty-nine.

Although I am a physician—a dermatologist—I knew little more about breast cancer than what I had learned in medical school in the late 1970s. Back then, I saw several patients who died from the disease, and I was afraid. So I started doing the "right things." I dutifully saw my physician every year for an exam (right). I had a baseline mammogram between ages thirty-five and forty (right) and a mammogram every other year between forty and fifty (right). I began planning for annual mammograms when I was about to turn fifty (right—though experts now recommend annual mammograms after forty). I also practiced breast self-examination on a "regularly sporadic" basis (wrong). Like many women, I had "lumpy" breasts, making self-examination difficult to interpret. I relied on my physicians and mammograms to keep me safe (very wrong).

When I learned that I had breast cancer, I was disappointed that three doctors who had examined me many times had failed to recommend a biopsy—a test that takes a tissue sample and analyzes it for cancer. I was disheartened that mammograms had failed to detect my cancer. But more than anything, I was amazed at myself—that I had been so cavalier about the very precautions that could have diagnosed my tumor sooner: doing monthly breast self-exams without fail, and insisting on further tests on a lump that worried me. Denial is a powerful emotion.

Fortunately, my cancer had not yet spread when it was diagnosed, at least not that the existing technology could determine. The tumor was medium-size—2.2 centimeters, a little under an inch, in diameter.

Surgery is almost always recommended for breast cancer. I chose to have a mastectomy—surgery to remove the breast—followed by chemotherapy. Women with breast cancer are offered chemotherapy when their tumors are of a certain size or they are in a high-risk category for recurrence. "Adjuvant treatments" such as chemotherapy and drugs such as Herceptin can prevent or postpone a recurrence of the cancer and improve the chance of long-term survival.

The usual chemotherapy for early-stage breast cancer, while no picnic, is no longer the ordeal it used to be. Now there are drugs to help with nausea and fatigue, and to stimulate blood-cell production in the bone marrow—thereby helping to prevent infection and possibly detrimental treatment delays.

Of course, chemotherapy has turned wig-making into a real growth industry. Your bad-hair day lasts about nine months. My daughter, Gail, had a lot of fun playing with my wig—or, as we called it, "the muskrat." Actually, I learned to appreciate the ease with which I could wash my "hair"—swish it in a bowl of suds, rinse it, and hang it to dry. I also enjoyed snatching it off at stoplights on the hot drive home from work and chuckling at other drivers' startled expressions.

Going through surgery and chemotherapy mobilized me, and it was easy to focus on milestones: one-third done, half-way done—finished! My eyelashes returned, and before I knew it, I was ready to donate the muskrat to the American Cancer Society's wig bank. I could climb the hill behind my house without gasping for breath, and, finally, I went an entire day without thinking about breast cancer.

My days now, since chemotherapy, are as precious as the glimpse of a small garden behind a city brownstone. These are good days. They have shown me, in a poignant and powerful way, that life is best lived by us all, with or without cancer, in a state of radical trust. Trust, and trust, and trust some more. None of us knows the limits of our days, but we do know Who limits them. And that is all we need to know.

—*Suzanne Braddock, M.D.*

$\mathcal{W}$ind

I sit silent in the cold room, reading,
when softly, a stir outside calls me away. It is the wind,
moving the frozen oaks and evergreens, pushing the snow
across the ice on the lake.
It is a sound both great and small,
the breath of God over the land
the voice of creation,
giving life to this cold, barren landscape,
to my days of terror.
I feel the power embraced in that sound,
and joy in the force that is greater than I,
greater than cancer,
greater than all the pain in all the women.

—*Suzanne W. Braddock, M.D.*

1

Breast Cancer: An Overview

*Y*ou might think the terms "good news" and "breast cancer" don't belong in the same sentence—or even the same zip code. And in one way, you'd be right: A diagnosis of breast cancer is never good news.

But amazing things are happening in breast cancer prevention, diagnosis, and treatment, and the good news just keeps getting better. For example, since 1989, the death rate from this disease has declined more than 2 percent a year, even though the number of cases has gradually risen. More than 200,000 women are diagnosed with breast cancer each year in the United States. And the majority of women whose breast cancer is discovered early are cured.

Partly because of a surge in breast cancer awareness, more and more women are learning about this illness and about their own level of risk. The more they know, the more faithfully they practice self-examination, schedule mammograms, and take care of their health. In turn, more cases of breast cancer are detected early and the survival rate continues to rise.

You can see why every woman, regardless of her age, needs information about breast cancer—especially in the United States, where the breast cancer rate is among the highest in the world. If you have breast cancer, knowledge is the most potent antidote to fear and the best preparation for treatment. If you do not have breast cancer, knowledge is your strongest protection.

The best way to start learning about breast cancer is with an understanding of the healthy breast.

1

Breast Anatomy

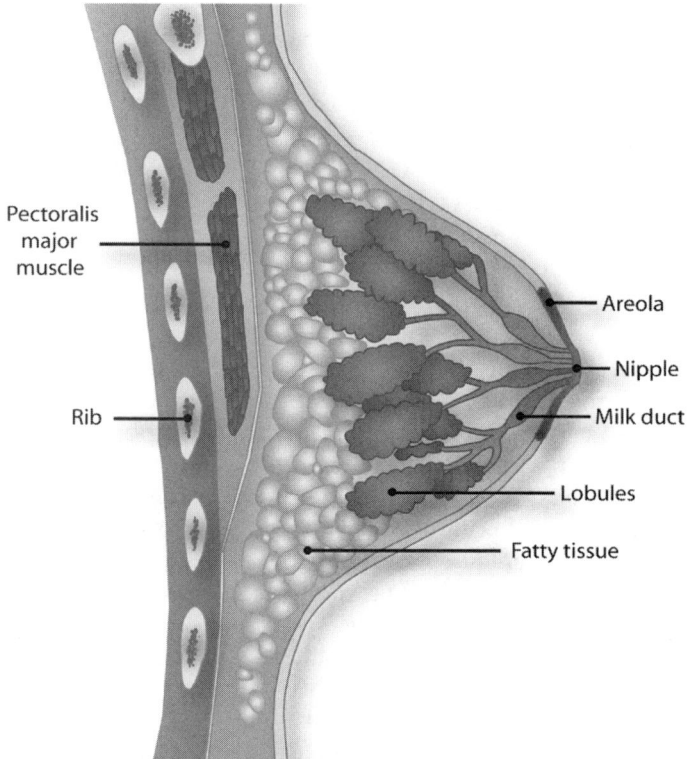

Breast Structure and Function

The human female breast is so glamorized and commercialized in our culture, it's easy to forget that the breast has a serious job—producing milk for babies. Even a quick look at breast structure reminds us of this important function.

The breast is made up of fatty tissue that contains blood vessels and lymph vessels, plus fifteen to twenty rounded divisions called *lobes*, themselves formed of dozens of smaller *lobules* that end in tiny *bulbs*. The lobular system produces milk in response to hormonal changes after childbirth or after an abortion or a late miscarriage. Milk flows from the lobes and bulbs through narrow tubes, or *ducts*, leading to the *nipple*, which protrudes from the center of the *areola*—the circle of darker skin at the tip of the breast.

Lymph vessels in the breast carry *lymph,* a pale fluid containing white blood cells, to *lymph nodes*—small, rounded masses of tissue that act as filters for this fluid. Lymph serves to transport infection-fighting cells to all parts of the body.

There are lymph vessels and nodes throughout the body, but the lymph nodes nearest to the breast are *usually* the first ones affected when breast cancer begins to spread. In a discussion of lymph nodes, you may hear the terms *sentinel node* and *axillary nodes.* The sentinel node is the first lymph node, in the underarm, that lymph fluid reaches. Axillary nodes refer to any of the lymph nodes in the armpit.

What Is Cancer?

Every part of your body, and of every other living thing, is made up of cells. In human beings, some cells divide to create new cells every twelve to twenty-four hours (unlike bacterial cells, for example, which can divide every twenty to thirty minutes). In the normal, orderly cell-renewal process, cells reproduce just fast enough to replace the ones that die off, keeping your blood and organs healthy.

When cells become abnormal and start to divide uncontrollably, the condition is called *cancer.* Eventually, an abnormal growth, or *tumor,* forms. Tumor cells not only act differently from normal cells, but they also look different under a microscope.

Breast cancer isn't a death sentence. We've made so much progress in the last twenty years. In the future, I believe breast cancer will be viewed more as a chronic disease, like hypertension or diabetes.
—Kathryn, oncology RN

Some tumors are *benign*—not cancerous. Benign tumors do not spread, so surgically removing them usually solves the problem. By contrast, a *malignant* (cancerous) tumor—if not detected and treated early—may spread from its original site to other parts of the body in a process called *metastasis.* Malignant tumors may be removed by surgery and treated with one or more additional types of therapy, depending on how large they are and whether they have metastasized.

Most breast cancers develop in the lobes or ducts of the breast. Scientists are still learning exactly how this occurs; they have identified certain risk factors—some proven, others more questionable. It is helpful to be aware of all risk factors.

Risk Factors for Breast Cancer

Hereditary Risks

Women in Western industrial countries have a higher risk of breast cancer even if they do not have a family history of breast cancer. In fact, most of the time—in about 70 percent of breast cancer cases—there is no known history of the disease in the woman's family. In such cases, the disease is called *sporadic* breast cancer. In another 20 percent of cases, at least one relative—more often an aunt or a grandmother than a mother or a sister—has had breast cancer. When this family history exists, the disease may be referred to as *polygenic* breast cancer. Even with a family history of polygenic breast cancer, many family members do not develop the illness.

I don't care how many breasts my mom has. I'm just happy she's okay.
—*Gail, 13*

In 5 to 10 percent of all breast cancers the disease is clearly passed from generation to generation, usually through genes BRCA1 (pronounced BRACK-uh 1) and BRCA2. Everyone has two copies of each of these genes, whose job is to repair cell tissues. So, it is not the genes themselves but the rare *mutations* (structural changes) in BRCA1 or BRCA2 that are responsible for truly *hereditary* breast cancer. But for these genes to give rise to cancer, both copies must have mutated.

A father or mother with one mutated gene, whether or not he or she develops cancer, has a fifty-fifty chance of passing the mutation to the next generation. Accordingly, a woman can have hereditary breast cancer while her mother and sisters stay cancer-free.

Approximately 55 to 65 percent of women who inherit a BRCA1 mutation will develop breast cancer by age seventy. About 39 percent of women with this mutation will develop ovarian cancer by age seventy.

At the same time, 45 percent of woman who inherit a BRACA2 mutation will develop breast cancer by age seventy, and 11 to 17 percent will develop ovarian cancer by age seventy.

More recently, cancer research showed that another gene, called PALB2, raises the risk of breast cancer in women nearly as much as the mutations in the BRCA1 and BRCA2 genes. Scientists found that women who had no family history of breast cancer but who had a mutation of the PALB2 gene, had a 33 percent chance of developing a malignancy by age seventy; women with the mutation *and* a strong family history of breast cancer had a 58 percent risk of developing the disease by age seventy.

Especially if you have a family history of breast cancer, talk to your doctor about genetic testing for *bilateral* breast cancer (cancer in both breasts). Most insurance plans, including Medicare, usually pay for genetic testing. It takes about three weeks, sometimes longer, to receive test results for BRCA1 gene testing; this information is helpful to both you and your physician in making decisions about breast surgery.

Environmental Risks

Every day, we are exposed to toxins in the form of pesticides, herbicides, cleaning solvents, chemical waste, food additives, certain plastics, and many other substances. Some are known *carcinogens* (cancer-causing agents). Others have been linked to higher rates of cancer among people exposed to them, but the cause has not been scientifically proven.

Hormonal Risks

Compared to the general population, a woman is at greater risk for breast cancer if she has been exposed to higher levels of *estrogen* over her lifetime. This exposure can be entirely natural, due to the factors listed below:

- early onset of menstrual periods (before age 12)
- late menopause (after 55)
- late first pregnancy (after 30)
- no pregnancies

Also contributing to lifetime estrogen exposure are medicines that contain estrogen, such as birth-control pills and drugs taken to ease menopausal symptoms. Most researchers doubt that the synthetic hormones in birth-control pills pose much of a breast cancer risk. Some studies suggest a slightly higher risk among long-term users of oral contraception and among women who started using them as teenagers.

Long-term estrogen-replacement therapy, during and after menopause, is a risk factor that diminishes when use of the hormone is stopped. Certain hormone combinations, however, are more carcinogenic than treatment with estrogen alone. These include estrogen and *progesterone* (or progestin, synthetic progesterone), which is sold under several labels, and estrogen and testosterone (usually sold as Estratest).

After my diagnosis, I dealt with anxiety by saying, "I'm alive today and will live today to the hilt." By fearing death, I figured I was dying all the time instead of living.
—Suzanne, 58

If you're taking a prescription drug for menopause symptoms, ask your doctor if it contains one of these combinations and, if so, whether you should switch to another drug.

DES (diethylstilbestrol), a synthetic estrogen, was prescribed from the 1940s until 1971 to prevent pregnancy complications. Women who took this drug have a slightly elevated breast cancer risk. Daughters who were exposed to DES in their mothers' wombs do not appear to share this risk, though it's impossible to be certain until more of these daughters reach their forties, fifties, and beyond—the ages at which breast cancer is more likely to occur.

Radiation Exposure

Women who have had radiation to the chest—perhaps as treatment for cancers such as Hodgkin's disease or for conditions such as tuberculosis or breast inflammation *(mastitis)*—are at greater risk for breast cancer. (Radiation as a treatment for nonmalignant diseases ended by the 1960s, once the risks were understood.)

If you have been treated with radiation to the chest, you should begin regular breast self-examination and annual mammograms no later than ten years after the radiation treatment

6

began. These precautions are all the more important if you were exposed during puberty, since developing breasts are especially vulnerable.

The small amount of radiation delivered in chest X-rays and mammograms are not a cause for concern—except possibly for women who have inherited mutated BRCA1 or BRCA2 genes.

Diet and Alcohol Use

If you are overweight, especially if you put on those excess pounds during adulthood, your risk is higher than other women's. The same is true if you drink alcohol. The more you drink and the younger you start, the higher the risk. As little as three alcoholic drinks a week increases the risk.

Nationality and Ethnicity

North America has one of the highest incidences of breast cancer in the world, followed by Western Europe, Australia/New Zealand, and Northern Europe. The incidence is lowest in China and central Africa. Genetic factors play a part, but environment and lifestyle may be equally important, since second- and third-generation immigrants to the United States are more likely to get breast cancer than their nonimmigrant relatives.

In the United States, white women are at slightly greater risk for breast cancer than African-American women, but the death rate is higher among African-Americans. The risk is lower among Native American, Hispanic, and Asian women.

Maintaining a positive attitude is very important as you go through the treatment. It may be the best medicine there is during breast cancer treatment.

—Jan, 69

Age and Gender

Clearly, a great many things carry some degree of risk for breast cancer, but the fact is, most women who develop the disease have not encountered any of them—apart from being female and getting older, neither of which you can do anything about. You can, however, do everything in your power to stay healthy and minimize your other risk factors. And you can—since no prevention measure is foolproof against breast cancer—spare no effort to find your cancer early if it should develop.

2

Getting a Diagnosis

You may tell yourself, "It's probably nothing"—that lump or thickness you think you feel in your breast. Perhaps you're thinking you should wait a while before going to see your doctor. Maybe you're thinking it really isn't a lump and that it will go away. Perhaps you're thinking about the fact that you're healthy and take care of yourself, so you shouldn't have breast cancer.

Still, it is important to investigate any suspicious change in your breast and schedule that mammogram and annual physical. Breast cancer tumors that can be felt are usually discovered by you or by your doctor during a routine physical. Most lumps that can't be felt show up in mammograms.

If you find a lump, the next step is to get it *diagnosed*—to find out whether it is caused by cancer or something else. Odds are, it's something else. Only about one out of five breast lumps is cancerous.

Methods of Examining the Breasts

Breast Self-Examination (BSE)

Many women discover their own cancers during a *breast self-examination (BSE)*. That's why every woman should examine her breasts every month. BSE should become routine as soon as the breasts develop, or by age twenty at the latest.

Because the breasts tend to swell during the menstrual period, premenopausal women should perform BSE three to five days after their period ends. Postmenopausal women should examine their breasts on the same day every month, so that the date itself is a reminder.

Some women, especially those in high-risk categories, avoid BSE because they are afraid of what they might find. This avoidance is understandable. It's also unhealthy, emotionally and physically. Frequent, habitual self-examination is by far the best way to discover a cancer while it is small and highly treatable, and finding a small tumor is much better than finding a large one.

My diagnosis was unbelievable to me. The radiologist kept saying she was concerned about my mammogram and I kept saying it was just scar tissue from a previous biopsy. Then it dawned on me that she was trying to tell me she thought I had breast cancer.
—Kristine, 51

One excuse some women use for not doing BSE is that their breasts are always lumpy—the result of normal, benign masses called *cysts* or *fibrocystic changes*. This condition is often mistakenly referred to as "fibrocystic disease," but it is not an illness.

If you chronically have benign masses in your breasts, you might assume that you wouldn't notice a new lump or one that is unusual. But if you examine your breasts regularly, you'll learn the "terrain." Once you're familiar with the texture and the pattern of cysts in your breasts, you will detect changes, even small ones.

Self-Examination Lying Down

Every month, use both BSE techniques: one lying down and one standing before a mirror. Lying down, you'll examine your breasts with your hands. To examine your breasts while lying down:

1. Place a small pillow under your right shoulder; then raise your right arm, and rest the back of your hand on your forehead. This position flattens the breast and makes it easier to examine.

2. Using the pads of the three middle fingers of your left hand, make small circular motions to examine your right breast with light, medium, and then firm

Possible Signs of Breast Cancer

During self-exams, watch for the following:

- a lump or thickening in the breast, surrounding area, or armpit
- swelling, redness, or rash
- puckering or dimpling of the skin
- skin texture like that of an orange (a condition called *peau d'orange*)
- itchiness, soreness, or scaling of the nipple
- drawing-in (retraction) of the nipple or another part of the breast
- unusual warmth that feels feverish in or near the breast
- any change in breast size, shape, or symmetry
- unusual pain in a part of the breast, armpit, or surrounding area
- bloody discharge from the nipple

pressure. Don't lift your fingers but keep them flat as you do this.

3. Use an up-and-down pattern, as if following narrow vertical stripes, to cover the entire breast and surrounding area-from collarbone to lower bra line to breastbone, and including the armpit.

4. Repeat steps 1 through 3 using the right hand to examine the left breast.

You can examine your breasts this way in the shower or bathtub, although if you're not lying down you lose the advantage of your breasts being flattened, which makes abnormalities easier to find. On the other hand, slick, soapy skin makes small changes more noticeable. You can get the soapy-skin effect while lying down by applying a smooth lotion or placing a piece of slippery fabric (such as satin) over your breast while you examine it.

Breast Self-Exam Lying Down

Lie down.
Place pillow under right shoulder.
Raise right arm above head.
Use the pads of the three middle fingers
of your left hand to examine your right
breast.

Examine area vertically from:
across the breastbone.
up to the collarbone
back to the armpit

Examine entire area.
Use vertical stripe pattern.
Use light, medium, and firm pressure.
Move fingers in dime-sized circles.
Repeat these steps using the right hand
to examine the left breast.

Self-Examination Standing in Front of Mirror

To examine your breasts in the mirror, look for any of the warning signs listed above. Do this in each of the following positions:

- with your arms down at your sides
- with both arms held straight up over your head
- with your hands pressed against your hips to tighten the chest muscles and bending forward at the waist

If you notice a warning sign during BSE, or at any other time, see your doctor. Don't put it off, and if the doctor's office staff tries to schedule your visit for "the next available appointment" six months from now, ask to speak with the doctor's nurse or with the doctor.

Do not assume that a lump can't be cancer if it moves (or doesn't move) or if it is hard (or soft), tender (or painless), or regular (or irregular) in shape. Any new lump or thickening should be examined by a doctor, regardless of its characteristics. If you are worried about a lump, insist on imaging studies (such as ultrasound or MRI) or a biopsy. You deserve a clear answer, and no doctor can provide one just by feeling the lump.

When I was diagnosed, tears came to my eyes, but I was more worried about my husband and two boys. How would they handle it if something happened to me? My main thought was helping them get through this.
—Julianne, 54

It is never safe to stop doing BSE. It should be a lifelong habit, even if you have had a mastectomy or lumpectomy. After surgery, begin examining the incision right away for changes, bumps, rigid areas, or discoloration, and search for lumps above and below the collarbone and in the armpit. Practicing BSE on the opposite breast is extremely important, too. Survivors of some types of breast cancer are at high risk for a new breast cancer in the opposite breast.

Breast Self-Exam in Front of Mirror

Arms at side.
Compare symmetry.
Look for changes in:
- shape
- color

Check for:
- puckering
- dimpling
- skin changes
- nipple discharge

Arms over head.
Check front and side view for:
- symmetry
- puckering
- dimpling

Hands on hips, press down, and bend forward.
Check for:
- symmetry
- nipple direction
- general appearance

Clinical Examination

Though a clinical examination is not a substitute for BSE, you should always have a clinical breast exam as part of your yearly checkup. Your doctor will feel the breasts and breast area for thickening or lumps, check for visible warning signs, and ask about breast tenderness or changes you might have experienced, your breast care, your medical history, and your family's medical history.

An experienced medical professional is usually more skilled than the patient at feeling the difference between a benign lump and a malignant one, but, as mentioned above, he or she can't be certain whether a lump or another symptom indicates cancer. If the clinical exam raises suspicions of cancer, further diagnostic tests will be needed. The most common ones are described below.

Mammography

Perhaps you've read or heard about the public debate over how soon a woman should begin having routine mammograms and whether or not mammograms are necessary for women in their forties. Please take note: The answer is yes they are! Mammograms save lives.

A *mammogram* is an X-ray of the breast—simple, widely available, and lifesaving. Scientists trying to understand why the number of breast cancer deaths fell 24 percent between 1990 and 2000 found that mammograms were the most important factor, followed by new ways of treating the disease.

Waiting for test results, for information, is the hardest. When you're afraid, any wait at all seems too long.

—Ann, 53

Having a mammogram takes only a few minutes. It's simply a matter of standing next to a mammography machine while a technician positions your breast on a small, square plate, compresses it against another plate, and takes the image. The process is repeated—two images for each breast—and all you feel is a brief pinch during the short time your breast is positioned between the plates.

Mammogram

A mammogram takes only a few minutes. It's recommended that women have their first mammogram between the ages thirty-five and forty. If you have a family history of breast cancer, talk to your doctor about a mammogram in your twenties.

The images are captured either on film, like a photographic negative, or on solid-state detectors similar to those in digital cameras. In the latter case, the image is called a *digital mammogram*. Digital mammography exposes the breast to even less radiation than a film mammogram, produces more detailed images, and more accurately depicts the comparatively dense breasts of younger women. Whichever type of mammogram you have, a radiologist will interpret the images and you'll learn the results in a few days. Ideally, the same radiologist will read all your mammograms and compare your most recent images with your older ones.

Mammograms are done for either screening or diagnostic purposes. A *screening mammogram* searches for early cancers that cannot be felt, while a *diagnostic mammogram* inspects a breast lump that can be felt or an abnormality detected in a screening mammogram. If you or your doctor finds a lump in your breast, a diagnostic mammogram is usually the next step.

3-D Mammography

3-D mammograms provide a better view of breast tissues. Key studies show that 3-D mammograms have increased the detection of invasive cancers by approximately 40 percent and all breast cancers by 29 percent.

A newer technology, known as *digital breast tomosynthesis,* is a screening test that allows doctors to examine breast tissue more thoroughly. Also referred to as a *3-D mammography,* it creates three-dimensional pictures of the breast with Xrays.

Research shows that the tomosynthesis along with traditional digital mammography detects up to 40 percent more invasive cancers and decreases false-positive rates by 15 percent. A *false positive* refers to a diagnosis of cancer when there is none.

If your breasts are healthy as far as you know, ask your doctor when to start having regular screening mammograms and how often you should have them. If you're in a high-risk category, she might want you to have your first mammogram while you're still in your twenties.

It is recommended that you seek out a certified breast center or clinic that offers digital mammography. By going to a certified facility, you can be assured that quality control measures are in place.

Sample Mammograms

A normal mammogram

Mammogram showing cysts with smooth edges

Mammogram with benign calcifications scattered throughout

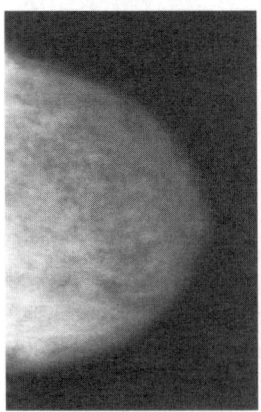

Mammogram showing a dense pattern, usually seen in younger women

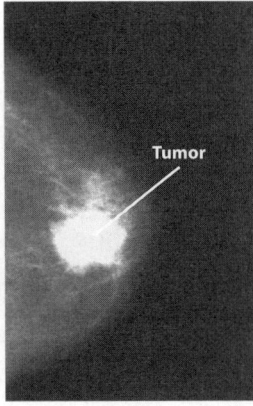

Mammogram showing cancerous growth. Note the irregular edges around the tumor.

Mammogram with cluster microcalcifications. These clusters are usually benign, but may be cancerous.

Breast Cancer in Men

Although it is rare, breast cancer does occur in men. Approximately 2,200 men between ages sixty and seventy are diagnosed annually. Symptoms include lump in the breast, nipple pain, inverted nipple, nipple discharge, sores on the nipple, and enlarged lymph nodes under the arm. Treatment for men is similar to that for women.

Screening for Breast Cancer

The following guidelines for breast cancer screening are recommended by several medical societies.

- A baseline mammogram, as a reference point to which future mammograms can be compared, when you are between thirty-five and forty
- An annual mammogram after age forty
- An annual mammogram if you have ever had breast cancer
- If your mother or sister has had breast cancer, an annual mammogram starting when you are ten years younger than the earliest-diagnosed relative. For example, if your mother developed breast cancer at forty-five and your sister at thirty-two, you should start having annual mammograms at twenty-two.

Don't be alarmed if your mammogram shows abnormalities and your doctor wants to do additional tests. Only 5 to 10 percent of "suspicious" abnormalities turn out to be breast cancer. False-positive results are so common that most women who have regular mammograms will eventually get that dreaded phone call or letter asking them to return for further tests, only to find that there is nothing wrong.

Be grateful for false positives, and for your doctor's diligence in following up on a suspicious abnormality that turns out to be harmless. The inconvenience and expense of follow-up diagnostic studies (usually another mammogram or an ultrasound) are easily outweighed by the many lives mammography saves, and by your peace of mind.

False-negative results are also possible, particularly in women with dense breasts. Mammography simply fails to "see" 10 to 20 percent of cancers in these dense tissues. Ask your doctor or your mammogram technician if you have dense breast tissue. If the answer is yes, your doctor may agree to order additional tests, such as ultrasonography, MRIs, or tomosynthesis.

Abnormal mammogram findings that must be investigated include:

- a white, starburst-shaped (spiculated) mass or nodule (as distinct from the clear, smooth edges of harmless cysts and benign tumors)
- uneven density (Dense areas in the breast are thicker than normal and whiter than the surrounding tissue. If these densities are larger in one breast, or appear in a different part of one breast than in the other, they may be cause for concern.)
- microcalcifications (calcium particles)—very common and usually benign, but if clustered in a certain way, might indicate cancer
- any change since your previous mammogram

In summary, get your first baseline mammogram between the ages of thirty-five and forty. If you have a family history of breast cancer, get your first mammogram ten years earlier than the age of your relative at the time of her diagnosis.

Ultrasonography

We have seen that mammography is a highly useful diagnostic test but is not foolproof. When both mammography and ultrasonography are used, a clearer picture can emerge.

Ultrasonography bounces sound waves off tissues and organs. The sound waves bounce back as patterns of echoes, which can be converted to images and projected onto a computer monitor. The procedure is painless, and you won't hear or see either the sound waves or the echoes.

To gather these images, an ultrasonography technician spreads a gel on your breast so that the sound waves can pass

---

When to Have MRI Screening for Breast Cancer

An MRI is recommended in addition to a mammogram if you:

- have a strong family history of breast or ovarian cancer
- have been determined to have a lifetime risk of breast cancer
- have dense breast tissue and a previous breast cancer was not detected by mammogram
- have had radiation to the chest between the ages of 10 and 30
- or a close relative has had any of these syndromes:

  — Cowden Syndrome—a rare disorder, causing noncancerous tumors on the skin or in the lining of the mouth and nose

  — Li-Fraumeni Syndrome (LFS)—a hereditary predisposition to cancer

  — Bannayan-Riley-Ruvalcaba Syndrome (BRR)—an uncommon condition, causing noncancerous polyps of the small and large intestines

MRI guidelines are from the American Cancer Society.

---

through more easily. Then he or she will pass a microphone-like device, called a *transducer,* over your skin. The transducer both emits the sound waves and transmits the echoes to the computer.

According to some researchers, mammography plus ultrasonography can find about 17 percent more tumors than mammography alone. Sometimes, ultrasonography can detect whether a lump in the breast is filled with fluid and most likely is a cyst, or if it is solid tissue that might or might not be cancer.

Magnetic Resonance Imaging (MRI)

Magnetic resonance imaging (MRI) uses powerful magnets and radio waves to produce computer images of selected body tissues. Among other things, these images reveal the blood vessels in different types of tissue. Cancer spreads by forming new blood vessels, so cancer tissues are often highly vascular, containing a great many more blood vessels than normal tissues.

Hundreds of images are taken, each representing a thin slice of tissue. A computer combines the images, which are read and interpreted by a radiologist.

If you are having MRI to detect breast cancer, you will probably be injected with a dye that is absorbed more quickly by cancerous tissue—where more blood vessels cluster—than by normal tissue or benign tumors. The radiologist will look for concentrations of this dye that might suggest a malignancy.

MRI can be an extremely useful and accurate diagnostic tool. False-positive and false-negative results are possible, of course, as with any test. For example, some nonmalignant tumors are highly vascular and thus appear malignant on MRI. Likewise, slow-growing cancers with relatively few blood vessels may look like normal tissue and yield false-negative results.

MRI is painless but can be time-consuming (thirty minutes to two hours), tedious, and noisy. You'll have to lie still most of the time as your bed moves slowly through a large cylinder. Ask your doctor how long the MRI will take and whether you can listen to music or an audiobook through the headphones provided. If you're claustrophobic, your doctor will probably prescribe something to relax you without putting you to sleep.

Because MRI is expensive and is unavailable in many areas, it is not as commonly used as mammography or ultrasonography for detecting breast cancer. Insurance may cover MRI for lumpectomy candidates (in order to confirm that the cancer is confined to the tumor) and in cases where a strong family history of breast cancer exists or a mutated BRCA1 or BRCA2 gene is present.

Diagnosing with Biopsy

If other tests haven't ruled out cancer, you and your doctor will schedule a biopsy—an outpatient procedure in which cells, sample tissue, or an entire tumor is removed from the body for microscopic examination. Then, a *pathologist*—a doctor who diagnoses disease from tissue or blood samples—examines the sample under a microscope, and may perform other tests on it as well, to see if cancer cells are present.

It's important for the physician who performs your biopsy to remove ample tissue from the sites where cancer is suspected. A biopsy, properly performed, can give a precise diagnosis and is the only sure way to establish whether a lump is malignant. For a tumor to be pronounced benign, the clinical exam, the mammogram, and the biopsy must all agree on the finding. For a cancer diagnosis, the biopsy alone is conclusive.

You should insist on a biopsy for any persistent or questionable lump, regardless of your family medical history or level of risk. It is your right to do so, even if others try to convince you that a clinical examination is sufficient.

There are several types of biopsies. The one your doctor recommends may depend on the size and exact location of the lump, the number of suspicious areas in the breast, and your own preference. Asking questions ahead of time, such as the ones suggested below, may lessen any anxiety you may feel about your biopsy.

- Which type of biopsy should I have?
- Will I be awake during the biopsy?
- How much tissue will be removed?
- What tests will be performed on the tissue sample?
- What are the risks and possible side effects of my biopsy?
- When and where will I learn the results and who will report them to me?

Diagnostic Biopsies

The three major types of biopsies are *fine-needle aspiration, core (large-needle) biopsy,* and *surgical biopsy.* Most biopsies are performed using a local anesthetic, which numbs the area from which the sample will be taken. Occasionally, more extensive biopsies are done with the patient under anesthesia.

Fine-needle aspiration (FNA) is the least invasive type of biopsy. It is used when lumps can be easily felt and located. The FNA procedure removes a small sample of cells through a narrow, hypodermic-type needle. Your doctor will insert the biopsy needle into the lump or thickening, then draw fluid into the syringe. A *cytologist* (a specialized pathologist who examines cells, rather than tissue or blood, for the presence of disease) then examines this fluid in the laboratory. If no cancer cells are found, your doctor may double-check the results with a more extensive biopsy, withdrawing a larger sample from the lump.

The biopsy preferred by many doctors is the large-needle or core biopsy. This biopsy takes a small, cylindrical sample of tissue from the lump rather than withdrawing only fluid. If the lump can be felt, the biopsy needle is inserted directly into it, without computer guidance. If the doctor can't feel the lump, he or she will use computer imaging or ultrasonography to guide the needle to the lump. This type of procedure is referred to as *image-guided* or *stereotactic core biopsy.*

> *Cancer brings so many issues to the table—sexual, financial, school, parenting, work. A couple who works together through these issues, which normally would be experienced over a longer period of time, will be brought closer together.*
> *—Holly, oncology social worker*

Other types of biopsies include the *Mammotome* (or *vacuum-assisted*) biopsy, which is a core biopsy that uses a larger tube, with the help of suction, to withdraw more breast tissue than in a traditional core biopsy.

An *advanced breast biopsy instrumentation (ABBI)* also withdraws a larger sample, using a rotating circular knife to excise the tissue. Some feel it is preferable to get a needle biopsy rather than an open surgical biopsy, since a needle biopsy does not disrupt the field for a later sentinel node biopsy, should one be necessary. As you may recall, the sentinel node is the first node that lymph fluid reaches after passing through the breast. (*See* page 55 for details on sentinel node biopsy.)

A negative core biopsy—one that shows no evidence of cancer—may or may not be conclusive. If there is a strong suspicion of cancer, based on an earlier imaging procedure or clinical exam, your doctor might schedule a surgical biopsy. But if a newly detected tumor "feels benign," and looks benign in imaging tests, then a negative core biopsy will be seen as confirming this assumption, and surgical biopsy will be unnecessary.

Surgical or open biopsy removes, through an incision, all or part of a lump or suspicious area for examination by a pathologist. *Incisional biopsy* involves removal of a tissue sample large enough for the pathologist to make a confident diagnosis, and the results of this procedure are usually conclusive. *Excisional biopsy* is, in essence, a lumpectomy—the entire lump and a small amount of the healthy tissue surrounding it are removed. Your doctor may choose excisional biopsy for small tumors that show no indications of spreading. If cancer is present, it will thus be removed in this single procedure.

Test Results and Tumor Characteristics

Waiting anxiously for the results can be the worst part of a biopsy, so ask your doctor when and how you'll learn your diagnosis. At the time of your biopsy, you might want to schedule a post-biopsy appointment with your doctor to discuss the results. It's up to you. If you do have breast cancer, would you prefer to get the news in person, with a relative or a friend there to support you? The alternative might be to wait for a phone call that could come at any time and under undesirable circumstances.

If the biopsy is positive, the combined results of all your diagnostic tests will show the characteristics of the cancer and will help your physician decide on the best course of treatment.

Size of the Tumor

Small tumors measure up to two centimeters (less than an inch) in diameter. Medium-size tumors are between two and five centimeters (up to two inches), and large tumors are more than five centimeters (two inches).

Presence of Cancer Cells
in Blood Vessels or Lymph Vessels

Because blood and lymph fluid circulate throughout the body, they can carry cancer cells almost anywhere. Thus, cancer cells in the blood vessels or lymph vessels signify a greater likelihood of metastasis (spreading0 to other parts of the body.

Appearance of the Cancer Cells

As normal cells mature, they take on distinctive, specialized shapes, depending on their function. Mature breast cells look very different from, say, mature skin cells or liver cells.

Well-differentiated breast cancer cells are typical of slow-growing cancers. They look much like normal, mature breast cells, with clearly defined boundaries. Very different in appearance are *poorly differentiated* breast cancer cells which have indistinct boundaries. These immature cells are found in aggressive tumors.

Hormone Dependency

The female hormones *estrogen* and *progesterone* are largely responsible for a woman's reproductive functions, including lactation (milk production in the breast). These hormones circulate throughout the body but interact only with cells that have special receptors where the hormones can attach themselves.

These hormones interact with cells in more than one way. Estrogen, for example, sometimes stimulates cell growth and sometimes blocks it. In the case of cancer, it is important to know which role estrogen plays. This can be determined by examining cancer cells to see which kind of hormone receptor, if any, is present. Testing cancer cells for estrogen and progesterone receptors can help doctors understand how aggressive the cancer might be and what kinds of therapy would be most effective.

Genetic Factors

Every invasive breast cancer should be tested for the HER2/neu (also called c-erB-2) receptor. HER2, short for "human epidermal growth factor receptor 2," is a gene—one of the thousands of genes that make up chromosomes and control the structure and activity of every cell in your body. They do this by producing, or "expressing," specific proteins to do specific jobs. The HER2 gene expresses the HER2/neu protein.

In 20 to 30 percent of breast cancers, the cells have more than two copies of this gene and express too much HER2/neu. The more copies of the gene there are, the more the protein is overexpressed and the more quickly the cancer is likely to grow.

Your doctor may also test the tumor for mutation of the *p53 gene* and schedule a *Ki-67* test. The p53 gene is normally a tumor suppressor that helps regulate cell growth; thus, an abnormal p53 gene can indicate uncontrolled cell growth. Ki-67 is a protein whose growth rate in cancer cells can be measured to reveal how fast a tumor is growing.

When I walk into a breast cancer patient's hospital room and tell her I am a ten-year survivor, I can see how good that makes her feel. I remember when I was lying in my hospital bed, I didn't think anyone survived.

—Dianna, 44

A K-67 test is now evaluated in pre-and post-therapy (chemotherapy or radiation) to determine early whether treatment is effective or needs to be changed.

You may find yourself exhausted by what seems like a never-ending barrage of tests. Understanding why your doctor orders a particular test and what information it provides may help you keep it all in perspective.

Testing for Risk of Recurrence

Whether or not a cancer spreads depends partially on the behavior of genes within the tumor. Thanks to technology, newer tests are now available to examine the genes of breast cancer tissue. These tests serve as indicators of whether a woman's risk of recurrence is low or high. Accordingly, the test results help doctors and patients choose the best line of postsurgical treatment. For example, if the risk is low, doctors may recommend hormone therapy. If the risk is high, doctors may recommend a more aggressive treatment that includes chemotherapy.

One such genetic test, *MammaPrint*, is used to evaluate tumor tissue. This test assesses seventy-one genes and determines the likelihood of cancer recurring within five to ten years of the initial diagnosis. *MammaPrint* can be used to test women under age sixty who have stage I or stage II breast cancer with negative nodes and tumors no larger than five centimeters (two inches).

Another test, *Oncotype DX,* provides information for postmenopausal women with early-stage (stage I or II), lymph node negative, estrogen receptor-positive breast cancer. The test assesses twenty-one genes and indicates whether a woman is at low or high risk for recurrence.

Types of Breast Cancer
Ductal Cancer
The most common form of breast cancer, ductal cancer starts in the cells that line the milk ducts. Between 70 and 80 percent of breast cancers begin in the linings of these tube-like tissues, whose purpose is to transport milk from the milk-producing lobes to the nipple during breast-feeding.

When abnormal cells are present but have not spread through the walls of the milk ducts, the condition is called *ductal carcinoma in situ,* or *DCIS. In situ* means "in the original place." DCIS is considered *preinvasive* because the abnormal cells are malignant and capable of becoming *invasive,* spreading into surrounding breast structures and beyond. For this reason, the first treatment for DCIS is surgery, either lumpectomy or total mastectomy.

Invasive ductal cancer usually is found in a single site, not at several locations throughout the breast or in the opposite breast. The overall risk of *bilateral* ductal cancer (that is, ductal cancer in both breasts) is only 0.8 percent per year after the initial diagnosis.

A DCIS lesion occasionally feels like a lump or a thickening of the duct, but it is more commonly detected first on a screening mammogram, where it can show up as a small cluster of calcium deposits called *microcalcifications*. Unfortunately, only about 50 percent of DCIS cases develop microcalcifications that can be seen on a mammogram. If cancer is suspected but is not visible on a mammogram, your doctor may use ductal lavage to flush out cells from the milk-duct lining. These cells are then analyzed for cancer. Otherwise, a DCIS lesion may be discovered incidentally, when a biopsy is performed on a breast lump, or go undetected until it becomes invasive.

Lobular Cancer

About 10 percent of breast cancers are *lobular carcinomas*. Lobular cancer begins in the milk-producing lobules and may become invasive, spreading into surrounding breast tissue.

Lobular carcinoma is less common than ductal cancer, but has the potential to affect both breasts more than other types of breast cancer. In about 30 percent of cases, this cancer is found in both breasts; it typically feels like a thickening in the breast in the area from the nipple to the underarm. Sometimes, the skin will pucker. Lobular carcinoma does not usually show up on a mammogram. An MRI scan is recommended in cases of lobular cancer to make sure all the sites are detected.

I highly recommend going to a breast cancer support group. You learn the tricks of the trade, hints for coping. No one really understands unless they've been through it.

—*Mary, 43*

Lobular carcinoma in situ (LCIS) refers to the presence of abnormal cells in the lobes. LCIS cells are not malignant, and the cells themselves do not develop into invasive cancer; however, these abnormal cells are signals of a risk that either lobular or ductal cancer will develop in either breast or both.

LCIS is rarely visible on a mammogram and is usually found during a biopsy on a breast lump. Treatment is either bilateral mastectomy or close observation. In some cases, LCIS is treated with the drug *tamoxifen,* which has been shown to prevent breast cancer in many high-risk women.

Other Breast Cancers

There are several less common types of breast cancers, each accounting for only about 1 to 1.5 percent of all breast cancers. The prognosis varies among these rare cancers.

Inflammatory breast cancer is an aggressive form of the disease that is often overlooked or misdiagnosed as infection. There is usually no lump to draw attention to inflammatory breast cancer. Rather, the cancer tends to be *diffuse,* or scattered—beginning in the ducts, spreading rapidly through the lymph vessels beneath the skin, eventually blocking the flow of lymph, and sometimes spreading along the chest wall. When symptoms appear, the breast may swell, feel warm or unusually painful, and take on a reddish tinge. The skin texture may change, developing ridges or thickening. When the skin looks pitted like the outside of an orange, the condition is known as *peau d'orange.* (Peau is French for skin.)

I felt so afraid after my diagnosis, even ashamed, because breasts are so personal. My first reaction was to hide and not let anyone know. But it helped so much to talk to someone. Talk to other women who have been through it.
—Billie, 48

Other warning signs of inflammatory breast cancer include:

- a mark like a bruise that does not go away
- nipple retraction
- bloody discharge from the nipple
- itching that isn't relieved by creams or ointments
- swelling in lymph nodes under the arm or above the collarbone

Warmth or pain in the breast, redness, and swelling are symptoms of breast infection, or *mastitis,* for which antibiotics are typically prescribed. When antibiotics don't clear up the problem, the next step is usually a biopsy.

Staging System for Breast Cancer

Primary Tumor (T)
TX: tumor isn't found or can't be measured
T0: no evidence of primary tumor
Tis: cancer *in situ* (has not grown into the breast tissue)
T1-T4: tumor size and/or extent it has grown into the breast tissue

Regional Lymph Nodes (N)
NX: nearby lymph nodes not found or can't be measured
N0: no evidence of cancer in nearby lymph nodes
N1-N3: size, location, and/or the number of lymph nodes involved

Distant Metastases (M)
MX: metastases not found or can't be measured
M0: no evidence of distant metastases
M1: evidence of distant metastases

Inflammatory breast cancer is a highly aggressive and dangerous form of the disease. Thus, it requires aggressive and immediate treatment, often in the form of chemotherapy followed by surgery, radiation therapy, additional chemotherapy, and hormonal therapy. If you have any inflammatory breast cancer symptoms, by all means see your doctor immediately and insist on a biopsy without delay.

Stages of Breast Cancer

Once your doctor knows exactly where the cancer is, additional tests will determine its *stage*—in other words, whether it has been caught early, late, or somewhere in between. Three characteristics determine the stage of a cancer: its size, its aggressiveness, and its location in sites other than the original tumor. The likelihood of disease-free survival (the patient's *prognosis*) can depend on the stage at which the cancer is diagnosed.

In 2003, the American Joint Committee on Cancer (AJCC) revised its breast cancer–staging guidelines. One reason for the change was the introduction of sophisticated tools such as *sentinel node biopsy,* whose ability to detect even small numbers of cancer cells made it possible to stage breast cancer more accurately. As a result, sentinel node biopsy has become the standard staging procedure for breast cancer, though it is by no means the only one.

Doctors use a variety of tests for cancer staging—a blood test for liver metastases, for example; a chest X-ray for metastases to the lung; or a PET/CT scan to gather additional information about the disease at the cellular level. At the time of cancer surgery, the doctor may withdraw bone-marrow cells to be examined for evidence of micrometastases, free-floating cancer cells that have not yet formed a mass.

Staging Guidelines

The AJCC staging guidelines identify tumors in three ways:

- size of the original tumor (T)
- lymph node involvement (N)
- metastasis (M)

A pathologist combines the characteristics of these three elements listed above—tumor size, lymph node involvement, and metastasis—to assign an overall stage for the cancer. The range of these stages is 0, I, II, III, IIIA, IIIB, IIIC, or IV.

The AJCC's 2003 revisions in breast cancer–staging guidelines allow more precision in staging—stage IIIC, for example, didn't exist under the old guidelines. One effect of the new guidelines has been *stage migration:* A cancer formerly identified as stage II, for example, might become a stage III cancer under the newer guidelines, though the cancer itself would not have changed. Many studies are underway as scientists try to learn whether the newer staging guidelines are indeed more accurate, whether they help doctors develop more effective treatment plans, and, ultimately, whether they save lives.

The chart on the following page is a general characterization of breast cancer at each stage. In the stage IIA and IIB descriptions, the phrase "microscopic disease in internal mammary nodes" refers to cancer found through sentinel node biopsy.

Breast Cancer at Each Stage

Stage	T	N	M	Description
Stage 0	*in situ*	0	0	DCIS or LCIS
Stage I:	1	0	0	Tumor 2 cm or smaller; no spread or metastases
Stage IIA:	0-1	1	0	No tumor, or tumor 2 cm or smaller, with cancer in 1 to 3 axillary lymph nodes or microscopic disease in internal mammary nodes; no metastases; or
	2	0	0	Tumor 2 to 5 cm; no spread or metastases
Stage IIB:	2	1	0	Tumor 2 to 5 cm with cancer in 1 to 3 axillary nodes or microscopic disease in internal mammary nodes; no metastases; or Tumor larger than 5 cm; no spread or metastases
	3	0	0	
Stage IIIA:	0-2	2	0	Tumor smaller than 5 cm with cancer in 4 to 9 axillary nodes or in internal mammary nodes; no metastases; or Tumor larger than 5 cm with cancer in 1 to 9 axillary nodes or internal mammary nodes; no metastases
	3	1-2	0	
Stage IIIB:	4	0-2	0	Tumor has grown into chest wall or skin; cancer in 0-9 axillary nodes; no metastases
Stage IIIC:	0-4	3	0	Tumor of any size; cancer in 10 or more axillary nodes or to other nodes on the same side; no metastases
Stage IV:	0-4	0-3	1	Tumor of any size has mestastasized to distant site.

3

Coping Emotionally

$\mathscr{I}$f you're like most women, when you heard the words "breast cancer," you may have thought you were going to die. Perhaps you have memories from years ago about family members or friends who did die from the disease. But, thanks to medical advances, this much-feared disease is no longer equated with imminent death. Although it is a life-threatening disease, breast cancer has become a treatable form of cancer, and many women who develop it are living long lives.

Meanwhile, it's normal to feel a barrage of emotions upon receiving a diagnosis. Shock, fear for yourself, fear for your family, denial, and panic are all common reactions. Suddenly, you have to gather and absorb a great deal of information you never dreamed you'd need.

Sometimes you may feel overwhelmed. But you will learn to manage these new demands and to honor your feelings. You will develop strategies for coping. Soon, your own, unique style of coping will become part of the wisdom breast cancer patients are eager to share; sooner than you think, you'll be helping others down the road you're traveling today.

Find Support

Studies indicate that the diagnostic phase is an extremely stressful time for women with breast cancer. Experts say talking with others about an illness helps to relieve some of the stress. Some women turn to their significant others, relatives, or close friends. However, there are a number of other ways you can find support that will help you through this worrisome time in your life.

Meet with Your Doctor

Your primary care doctor—the one you see for routine health care—may be an excellent initial source of information. Make an appointment to see him or her as soon as possible after your diagnosis. Here are some tips for your first appointment:

- Write down all your questions. Give a copy to the doctor and keep one for yourself. That way, you won't be tempted to skip some of the questions if you feel you're taking up too much of the doctor's time.
- Do some research on your own before your appointment if it eases your mind. The more you know beforehand, the more new information you can absorb during your conversation.
- Don't expect to be on top of things right away. There's a lot to learn.
- Invite your mate or a close friend to go with you. Your mate can take notes and help you remember the discussion in detail.

Conduct Your Own Research

Not all your questions about breast cancer will be answered during the first meeting with your doctor. New questions will come up. Jot them down as they occur to you. Books, articles, and websites offer vast amounts of information, from the general to the specific.

Familiarize yourself with the library, local bookstores, and the Internet. You'll find dozens of books on breast cancer, ranging from the very technical and scientific to simple presentations of pertinent facts. Decide how much you want to know and then look for publications that will meet your needs.

If you have access to the Internet, you'll find thousands of sites that publish material online, offer books and pamphlets for sale, or both. You'll also find breast cancer organizations, chat rooms, support groups, and inspiring stories of other women who have, or have had, breast cancer. These can be enormously comforting and helpful to you at every phase of dealing with the disease. If you don't have a computer or you're unfamiliar with the Internet, most libraries have public computers and staff who can show you how to use them.

Questions to Ask Your Physician

- What kind of breast cancer do I have?
- Will I lose my breast?
- What are my chances for long-term survival?
- Are further tests needed to find out whether the cancer has spread?
- How will I know which course of treatment is best for me?
- When will I begin treatment?
- How long will it take to recover from surgery and other treatments?
- Can you suggest support groups or services that might help me and my family?

Be careful about the websites you visit. Not all are accurate and up-to-date. Make sure the site sponsor is reputable. If you come across confusing or conflicting information, ask your doctor about it.

Meet with a Survivor

Breast cancer survivors say that one of the most important things you can do for yourself is meet face-to-face with at least one woman who has been successfully treated for breast cancer. Find someone who has a positive attitude and who is a good listener. You might already know someone who fits that description, or your doctor can refer you to patients he or she has treated. Online conversations are well and good, but your computer can't give you a hug, hand you a Kleenex, or hold your hand.

Minimize Outside Obligations

Life goes on, even if you aren't able to in your usual fashion. Some women continue with all their activities during breast cancer treatment; others decide to scale back a little, or a lot. You may need to rethink your professional and community responsibilities. If you serve on committees or boards, or lead a scout troop, or volunteer at a homeless shelter, let people know if you need to be out of commission for a while and that someone else will have to fill in for you.

At your job, try to anticipate problems and prepare for them. Work with your employer to find a temporary replacement for the times you can't be there. Check to see how much sick leave you can take, what your employer's extended-leave policy is, and whether you have long-term-care insurance. You might not need a long absence from work, but it's good to know how to arrange one if necessary.

If your employer is uncooperative, remember that state laws and the federal *Americans with Disabilities Act* and *Family Medical Leave Act* exist to protect your job, your benefits, your seniority, and your status, and require your employer to provide "reasonable accommodation" to you during your treatment and recovery. These laws apply to most public agencies and all but the smallest private employers. (Some federal employees are covered by a different law.)

For details on your legal rights under state and federal law and to receive an informative booklet, contact the American Cancer Society (*See* the Resources section at the back of the book).

Be Involved in Your Treatment

The level of your involvement in your treatment really is up to you. The questions that are most important to you, and your urgency in getting them answered, will serve as a guide. Bit by bit, you'll discover whether you want detailed information about every procedure, medication, and treatment option, or whether you're content to know only enough to be an informed patient.

Take your time deciding how involved you want to be—then feel free to change your mind. Maybe at first you'll want to be a walking breast cancer encyclopedia, but later, after getting to know and trust your cancer specialist, decide you are satisfied with just a grasp of the general principles.

Seek Emotional and Psychological Support

Think about coping strategies that have helped you keep your balance in the past. You can rely on this inner strength now. But if your coping skills aren't up to the task, your doctor, your research, and your support system can help.

It's natural to experience powerful and sometimes conflicting emotions after a diagnosis of breast cancer. Acknowledge your feelings and give them room. Confide in people who will listen and understand—even when your feelings are difficult to describe—and avoid well-meaning friends who try to talk you out of feeling the way you do.

Do not deny your emotions, no matter how inappropriate they might seem at first. Who knows? Tuning in to your most turbulent emotions, and surrendering to quietly pensive feelings as well, might surprise you with moments of great joy, even in the midst of sorrow and anger. Life warrants all these feelings, and more, and a crisis such as breast cancer can bring all of life into sharp focus.

I feel like I've been able to help others through my own breast cancer. All of my co-workers had mammograms right after I was diagnosed. One of them found she had a malignancy in the very early stages.
—Joan, 47

Your goal of feeling strong and at peace is not well served if you explode in anger over small things, take your fears out on others, or pretend to be on top of things when you're not. As with most situations, a balanced and honest approach is the most effective.

Find creative ways to uncover and release your emotions. Writing, making music, dancing, drawing, painting, doing home-improvement projects, gardening, and even cooking can be excellent ways to express your feelings and create something worthwhile in the process. Conversation—intimate, confidential talk with your husband, partner, or a friend—can be healing and strengthening if that person is supportive.

If your emotions seem out of control, however, and nothing has helped, consider getting professional counseling. Ask your doctor to refer you to someone who specializes in working with cancer patients, especially women with breast cancer.

Strong emotion is not inappropriate. Tears and anger are normal and even healthy ways to keep from bottling up your feelings. Allow yourself to cry and grieve. Give yourself permission to be angry. As long as your anger isn't unleashed on them, the people who care about you should accept it and not scold you for "giving in to it." The most uncomfortable feelings of sadness and anger will be resolved sooner if you plod on through them rather than try to sneak around them.

Choose the appropriate time and place to punch pillows or shout yourself hoarse. Let your anger become the energy that pushes you to learn, take charge, take care of yourself, hang on to humor, and hope. But if, instead of releasing your anger, you end up feeling angrier than ever, consider it a sign that you could benefit from counseling or a therapeutic support group.

You might think the feelings that surge inside you have never been experienced by anyone else. The truth is, you're not alone. Others have felt, or are feeling right now, the very same emotions.

Join Support Groups

Other breast cancer patients can offer you validation and hope. They can understand your feelings and experiences. In fact, your support group might become vitally important, if only to relieve your feelings of isolation. Knowing you are not alone can give you great comfort.

Breast cancer support groups are made up of women of all ages and from all walks of life. Most large hospitals offer support groups specifically for women with breast cancer. Those who take advantage of these groups report that the meetings and the new relationships give them strength. Hearing others express fears, celebrate triumphs (large or small), and share valuable information can be healing and calming. Sadly, the women who could profit most from a support group—those who are the most depressed, anxious, and fearful—often don't join one.

I had friends who had breast cancer and they really got me through the tough times. I would lay out all my fears and one of them would always have something funny to say about it. We would just howl. It's hard to be afraid of something when you can laugh at it.
—Ann, 53

The National Cancer Institute's Cancer Information Service, the American Cancer Society, and your hospital or breast cancer clinic can help you find appropriate support groups that meet face-to-face or online. The National Coalition for Cancer Survivorship helps cancer survivors and their families start local support groups or contact existing ones. For information about contacting these organizations, *see* the Resources section at the back of this book.

Examine Your Spirituality

Some women already have strong religious faith or spirituality when they learn that they have breast cancer, or they soon find themselves drawn toward greater spirituality. Others rely on their own grit and self-reliance to see them through.

If you are spiritually inclined, your experience with breast cancer could deepen your faith. Talking with a minister, rabbi, priest, or other spiritual adviser about your illness may offer comfort. It can also become an opportunity to learn more about what you believe, what you fear, and what your particular faith teaches about God, mortality, the self, and the most satisfying way to live.

Most of these questions concern everyone, whether or not they profess religious faith, so they are worth your contemplation. If you are not religious, talking with those who are can be enlightening. You can also find wisdom in the works of nonreligious thinkers and in poetry, art, literature, and nature. Finding ways to look beyond the boundaries of your own life—perhaps seeing order and purpose there—can bring you peace and comfort. It is the kind of comfort that comes from feeling yourself small—not smaller than others, just part of an immense and very grand universe.

When my mom first told me about her cancer, I was worried. Who would take care of me? What if she dies? She was totally honest with me. That was reassuring.
—Gail, 13

Practice Meditation, Good Nutrition, and Exercise

One way to quiet your mind and relieve your anxiety is to meditate. Spending just ten to twenty minutes, twice a day, in a deeply relaxed and focused state not only confers a sense of tranquility but also helps the body fight the damaging effects of stress.

Some women meditate by silently repeating the word "peace" while calmly releasing any distractions that arise in the mind. Others use a form of meditation called *visualization* or *guided imagery*. In a state of deep relaxation, they picture the body healing itself. They intently visualize their cancer shrinking, their immune cells fighting like microscopic armies against cancer cells, their energy returning, their color radiant, their life in balance.

If meditation appeals to you, learn more about it through your research on the Internet or in publications. Consider taking a class in meditation or yoga. Some styles of yoga use stretches, movement, and body postures to promote a meditative state. Others focus more on yoga as exercise. Either can calm and energize you. In fact, any activity that lifts your spirits and supports your overall health will improve both your mental and physical well-being.

Eating healthfully is another way to fight your cancer. A nutritious low-fat diet has been shown to decrease the risk of getting cancer. Raw foods believed to inhibit cancer growth include broccoli, cabbage, brussels sprouts, cauliflower, mustard greens, turnip greens, kale, and radishes. Animal studies have demonstrated that dietary fiber can reduce the risk of breast cancer, perhaps by preventing estrogen from stimulating the growth of breast malignancies.

Other studies suggest that a diet high in the antioxidant vitamins A and C, as well as beta carotene (which the body converts to vitamin A), offers protection against cancer.

Recent research has shown that vitamin D may provide protection from diseases such as cancer, osteoporosis, hypertension, and some autoimmune diseases. Ask your doctor about the dosage that is right for you.

More than a hundred studies have found significant decreases in cancer rates among people whose diets are high in the fruits and vegetables that contain these vitamins. Studies have not confirmed the benefits of taking vitamin pills.

Good sources of beta carotene are apricots, beet greens, black-eyed peas, cantaloupe, carrots, sweet potatoes, pumpkin, and spinach. Women with breast cancer who exercise have an improved outcome compared to those who do not. Further, women with breast cancer who exercised during treatment reported that they had more energy and did not gain as much weight as those who didn't exercise. Movement, swimming, and even dance or other programs can offer a physical and emotional boost.

Put Your Own Needs First

This really isn't as selfish as it sounds. In the long run, everybody will be better off because you took care of yourself when you needed to. Even so, it's difficult for many women to hand off their responsibilities. We are society's caretakers, its wives and mothers and usually its nurses, secretaries, child-care workers, and schoolteachers. We tend to put our loved ones' needs before our own. A breast cancer diagnosis can require a sudden reversal of lifelong habits, which at first, will likely be yet another source of stress.

Let people close to you be helpful. You don't have to be Superwoman. Explain to your family and friends that you must put all your energy into your treatment—not only surgery and therapies, but also learning, resting, and staying focused, which will help you keep your spirits up.

Addressing the Needs of Others

Throughout your treatment, you'll naturally be concerned about the people close to you. Putting yourself first doesn't mean ignoring your friends and family, especially your children. Though most of your active care for others should wait until your treatments have ended, there are ways to help without immersing yourself in their difficulties.

After working with breast cancer patients for fourteen years, I've found that patients connecting with other patients is the key to coping. Patients sharing their journeys is the best medicine.
—Ann, oncology social worker

As much as you want to spare your family and friends any pain, worry, or inconvenience, in one way or another your breast cancer will affect everyone around you. Your husband or life partner, especially, is likely to experience intense emotions. Your children's reactions will depend on their age, personality, gender, and stage of emotional development. Your friends, especially women close to you in age, will not only be concerned about you but might also be somewhat anxious, knowing that they, too, could develop breast cancer.

Some people will know instinctively how to comfort you and offer help. Most will not, at least at first. Some never will be able to. There is no "right way" for someone to react to your illness. Try not to judge or be hurt when friends or relatives are awkward around you or even avoid you. It doesn't mean they don't care. It's just that everyone copes differently and expresses emotions in different ways.

The following sections describe what the people in your life might be going through and how you can acknowledge their struggles without letting them wear you down.

Spouses

If your spouse is the strong, silent type, he may hesitate to discuss his feelings for fear of burdening you. He might go into denial about your disease, or he might overcompensate by being excessively cheerful. The more you share your feelings and needs with him, the better he may be able to face his own. You might need to give him explicit permission to open up emotionally. But perhaps he can't do that, or provide the support you need, no matter how much he loves you. Sometimes people just get mired in feelings of fear, sadness, anger, or helplessness in the face of their partners' disease.

For a whole year, I woke up each morning and said to myself, "You have breast cancer." It was like being on an emotional roller coaster.
—Kristine, 51

Letting him know that you don't blame him—and that you are not without support from friends, clergy, a counselor, or a support group—could help him deal with his own emotions. Eventually, he might learn how to help you by helping himself. Or he might not, in which case you can choose to accept him the way he is. The alternative—a constant, smoldering resentment—will be at least as harmful to you as to him.

Remind relatives and friends that they can make a world of difference by offering a kind word, babysitting, or otherwise sharing responsibility with your husband. Looking back, many husbands say they would simply like to have been asked, "How are you doing?"

If your husband, or anyone else, asks, "What can I do to help you?" take him up on the offer. Have him do something constructive—some activity that will reduce your anxiety.

Children

Children of every age, newborn to adult, are profoundly affected by a mother's breast cancer. Even infants are attuned to their parents' emotions and unsettled by the secrecy surrounding illness. The best thing you can do is accept their natural reactions to your cancer. Answer their questions with as much or as little information as they can absorb at their age and level of development. It might help them to confide in a trusted adult who isn't caught up in the crisis—a school counselor, teacher, neighbor, pastor, or friend.

Babies and Toddlers

The youngest children often respond to parents' stress by crying more, needing more attention, eating less, and sleeping poorly. Hold and comfort them as often as possible. Try to keep them on a consistent schedule. If they have begun to talk, give them very simple information ("Mommy's sick") and prepare them for changes in the household routine ("She might have to go away for a few days to get better").

Children Ages Three to Six

At these ages, children do not yet have reasoning skills and can see things only from their own point of view. They might think they caused the cancer or they might worry about getting sick themselves. Since young children tend to fear separation, prepare them for your absences. When neither parent can be with them, they should be cared for (preferably at home, where they feel safe) by someone they know well and trust.

Because they don't understand their emotions, they might act out—throwing tantrums, hitting, pushing, crying. Try to maintain their daily routine. Calmly, in simple terms, explain any changes from that routine. Comfort them, reassure them that they are not at fault, and acknowledge that they might feel sad or scared.

Children Ages Seven to Eleven

By these ages, children are beginning to think logically. Capable of reasoning, they are also capable of understanding (and fearing) the finality of death. They'll be most anxious about the immediate future, however. They might worry about the tangible effects of your cancer, such as the cost of medical care or the welfare of younger siblings. Acknowledge their fears and other feelings, and assure them that adults have these matters well in hand.

Always be truthful, without giving them more information than they can grasp. If you can't promise you'll recover, give them realistic reasons for hope, such as treatment advances, new discoveries through research, and inspirational stories about women who have beaten the odds.

Adolescent Children

From age twelve through their teenage years, children experience rapid physical, psychological, and emotional changes that make them extremely vulnerable. Because they are trying hard to establish their independence, develop their own identity, and separate from parents and childhood, they typically deny their vulnerability. Teenagers cling to self-absorption—the way a bud seems to hold itself tightly before it flowers—and think that bad things happen to other people, not to them.

Their mother's illness can undermine this certainty and draw them back into childhood and dependency. Be sensitive to this. Ask them to help out in tangible ways, recognizing that they are approaching adulthood but still have one foot in childhood. Talk about your own feelings in ways they can understand and deal with. This might prompt them to do likewise. But don't push. Sometimes, just being together is more reassuring than serious talk.

Adult Children

Your grown children will want to know how they can help, whether they live nearby or on another continent. No matter what their ages, a mother's serious illness can awaken long-forgotten feelings of dependence and deep anxiety, which may in turn trigger the need to control.

A son, for example, who typically uses his competence to deal with uncertainty might want to take charge of your care. Welcome his concern, share information with him, but firmly assure him that you are capable of making all the necessary decisions.

Daughters are likely to worry about their own susceptibility to breast cancer, as well they should. Emphasize the importance of monthly breast self-examination and annual checkups. Express the hope that your breast-cancer diagnosis will actually reduce their own risk by making them more conscientious about preventive care.

Other Family Members, Friends, and Acquaintances

Members of your extended family will naturally feel the impact of your cancer in different ways. Your parents may fear for you as they did when you were a child, and you might find your traditional roles turned upside-down as they look to you for comfort and reassurance.

Your siblings, besides being worried, will also feel a bit fragile themselves. If you are the first person of your generation to have cancer, they'll be awakened to their own vulnerability. If your cancer is hereditary, your sisters will have to confront their own breast cancer risk and that of their daughters. These concerns may seem selfish, but they also are quite realistic and they certainly don't diminish your siblings' love for you or their compassion for your struggle.

Family and friends will deal with your illness in ways that reflect their personalities, character, emotional makeup, and just plain busy-ness. Don't be offended by those who don't call or visit as often as others or who are less forthcoming with food, favors, and willingness to sit and talk with you. Some people have no idea what to do or say. Let them know that you understand, that it helps just to know they care, and that you're still interested in their day-to-day goings-on. Your reassurance might free them to show their concern more openly.

Maintain Sexuality and Intimacy

There's no medical reason to delay having sex after breast surgery unless your doctor advises otherwise. But you might not be particularly interested in sex right away, for a variety of reasons. For one thing, you've just had surgery and you'll be gathering your strength for a while. On top of that, your non-surgical therapy—radiation, chemotherapy, hormonal therapy, or another treatment—can temporarily dampen your desire, tire you, or cause other symptoms (such as vaginal dryness) that are likely to bump sexual activity off the top of your priority list.

After a mastectomy, with or without breast reconstruction, you have an entirely new body image to adjust to, and it will take some time for you to feel sexy and appealing. At the same time, you're fearing your partner's reaction to your altered anatomy, he might be reluctant to approach you for fear of causing you physical pain. But if you're not communicating, it's easy to draw the wrong conclusions, each of you perhaps thinking the other is indifferent.

For some couples, unacknowledged barriers to intimacy are a serious threat to the relationship. A discussion with your doctor might be helpful for the two of you. The doctor can explain to what extent your problem might be physiological, caused by treatment-induced hormonal changes, and to what extent it is emotional. He or she can reassure your partner that having sex won't cause you physical injury. And your doctor or a counselor can open the lines of communication between the two of you. Clearly, communication is crucial here. If the two of you don't share your fears openly, there's a lot of room for misunderstanding. Keeping quiet about anxieties will only push them deeper.

Assure your partner that you find him desirable. Tell him about your insecurities, and encourage him to share his feelings as well. Most husbands prove to be loving, supportive, and accepting of their wives' changed bodies and their topsy-turvy feelings.

My doctor found my breast cancer during a routine mammogram shortly after I turned 40. I immediately started to cry and thought I was going to die, but I didn't.

—Alice, 46

Until you are energetic and confident enough to have intercourse, you can maintain closeness by cuddling, holding, caressing, and confiding in one another. Without question, do not have sex until you're ready. Experts are unanimous on this point: Feeling obligated to have intercourse when you'd rather be doing almost anything else can be an ever-present source of stress and guilt feelings, which aren't beneficial at any time but can be especially harmful to you now. Allow time for your body and spirit to heal, and look forward to a lifetime of growing, changing, and maturing intimacy with the one you love.

4

Surgery for Breast Cancer

Virtually every woman diagnosed with breast cancer undergoes surgery, which may or may not be followed by radiation and other therapies. Today, women with breast cancer can choose from a variety of surgical options that were not available to their mothers. This is good news. Modern surgical techniques have increased survival rates and helped many women avoid losing one or both breasts. Yet the array of options can make it more difficult to weigh the relative advantages and disadvantages. Many women feel overwhelmed by unfamiliar medical terms and decisions to make at a time when they are already emotionally overwrought. They may feel their very lives depend on the right choice, and yet they also feel numb, unable to focus or make sense of things just when the need for clarity is great.

For this reason, it's a good idea to take your partner or a close friend with you when you first meet with your surgeon. Have your companion take notes or tape-record these conversations so that you need not grasp and remember all the new information laid out before you. Later, you and your companion can talk everything over.

Choosing a Breast Surgeon

After a breast cancer diagnosis, your doctor will likely refer you to a breast surgeon. If you like and trust the breast surgeon to whom your doctor has referred you, great! If not, perhaps you'll want to find the surgeon who is right for you. How do you go about this?

- Ask your physician for another referral.
- Get the names of breast cancer surgeons in your area from several credible sources: friends, co-workers, physicians, nurses, and other health professionals. Find out which of these surgeons are on the staffs of highly rated hospitals. Develop a working list, then look at the doctors' credentials on their websites. Interview as many as it takes to find one whom you trust and feel comfortable with.
- Get in touch with an organization such as the National Cancer Institute (NCI), the American Cancer Society, or the American Society of Breast Surgeons. Contact information for these and other organizations appears in the Resources section at the back of this book.
- Find breast cancer hotlines or women's health groups in your area that can point you toward breast cancer specialists and other resources.
- If you're involved in a support group or online chat room, ask other members how they went about their own searches.

Once you have found the right surgeon, he or she can refer you to other specialists, such as a radiation oncologist, who oversees radiation therapy, or a medical oncologist, who oversees any type of chemotherapy. As before, you don't have to accept the surgeon's recommendations and may wish to evaluate each doctor on your own.

In general, a doctor who is ethical, experienced, and attuned to your needs is one who:

- shows genuine concern for you and is not overly clinical or detached
- is a good teacher, explaining things thoroughly but clearly, in language you can readily understand
- takes a detailed history and performs a complete physical exam
- asks how you're feeling emotionally, who is helping you through your crisis, and whether you have or

need a support group

- gives you a realistic picture of your illness and outlook but is calm and reassuring
- has considerable experience with cases like yours
- is up-to-date on the newest treatments and research
- welcomes the involvement of family members or a close friend
- supports the use of all necessary pain control
- patiently answers all your questions and does not regard any of them as unimportant
- notices when you're confused or anxious and tactfully draws you out
- encourages you to get a second opinion on any treatment decision

Before Surgery

You will no doubt have questions about your surgery. When it comes to your breast cancer and its treatments, there's no such thing as an inappropriate question. Ask your doctor *before* you check in for surgery about anything that concerns you, though it might not be possible to answer some of your questions until after surgery. Here are some sample questions to help you start your own list:

- Will I need radiation therapy, chemotherapy, hormonal therapy, or targeted therapy following my surgery?
- When is breast reconstruction safer—at the time of surgery, or later? Which do you recommend?
- What side effects can I expect from surgery?
- Will my surgery be done on an outpatient basis, or will I be hospitalized? If so, for how long?
- Where will my surgical incisions be? What will my scars look like?
- Will I have drainage tubes?
- When will I be able to go back to work?
- Will my physical activities be restricted? For how long?
- Will I need physical therapy?

Discuss Surgical Incisions and Scars

Before your breast surgery, talk with your surgeon about the incision or incisions that will be used. If you are having a partial mastectomy, you will want to know how much scarring to expect and how the surgeon will keep scarring to a minimum. The shape and direction of the incision can influence whether your remaining breast tissue will pucker, whether your scar will draw the nipple out of its normal position or show above a bathing suit, and whether your breast will have any concave areas.

If your entire breast will be removed and you want to have reconstruction, ask how much of your skin can be spared for the process and how the incision will be positioned to allow for the best cosmetic outcome.

Techniques for hiding or minimizing scars are continually improving. For example, since the nipple position and weight distribution are completely different in upright positions, surgeons now decide on placement of incisions based on the appearance of a woman's breasts when she is standing, sitting, and walking, rather than during an examination, when she is lying down.

Types of Breast Surgery

The type of breast surgery your surgeon recommends depends on several factors, including the type, stage, and location of the cancer; your feelings about breast preservation or reconstruction; your prognosis; and your general health.

Overall, breast surgery is straightforward, and complications are rare. Hospital stays depend on the surgery being performed and whether any reconstruction will be done. Most stays are overnight; longer stays—two to six days—are sometimes needed if reconstruction is done immediately after the cancer surgery.

Partial Mastectomy

When a portion of the breast is removed during surgery, the procedure is called a *partial mastectomy*. There are two major types of partial mastectomy—*lumpectomy* and *quadrantectomy*. The difference between them is the amount of the breast that is removed. Partial mastectomies are usually outpatient procedures, even with lymph node removal.

For the preinvasive condition ductal carcinoma *in situ* (DCIS), partial mastectomy is often performed to remove the malignant cell clusters that are otherwise likely to invade surrounding tissues.

Confer with your surgeon about the advantages and disadvantages of lumpectomy and quadrantectomy in your situation.

Lumpectomy

Also known as *breast conserving therapy (BCT),* a lumpectomy removes the tumor and some of the surrounding healthy tissue. This procedure is possible when a tumor is small, easy to access, and situated so that a complete margin of healthy tissue can be taken and analyzed. The *margin* is the border of normal tissue remaining around the tumor that has been removed. A wide margin that is clear of cancer indicates that the entire tumor has most likely been removed and the chance of a local recurrence (cancer returning to the same site) is low.

Quadrantectomy

A *quadrantectomy* removes all or most of one quadrant of the breast, including the skin and connective tissue, and some- times the underarm lymph nodes. A quadrant, which represents about one-fourth of the breast, is not an ana-

Lumpectomy

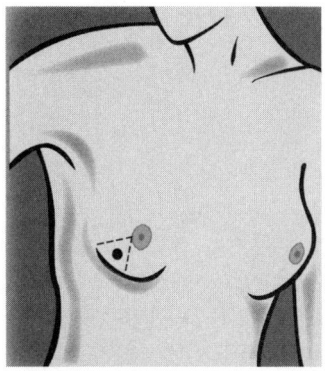

In a lumpectomy procedure, the lump and surrounding tissue are removed.

Quadrantectomy

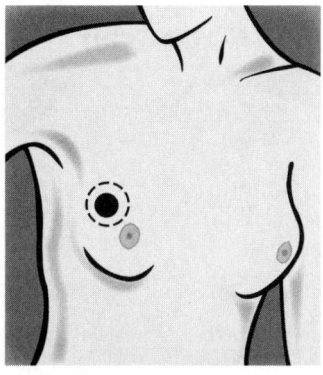

When performing a quadrantectomy, the surgeon removes the tumor, some surrounding breast tissue, and the lining over the chest muscles.

Total Mastectomy

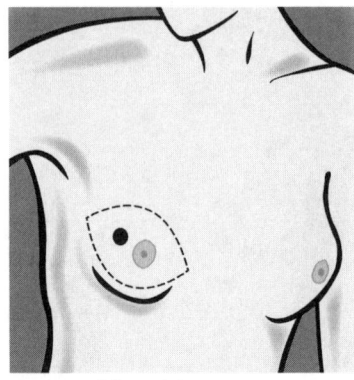

In a total (simple) mastectomy procedure, the entire breast is removed, but no lymph nodes are removed.

Modified Radical Mastectomy

A modified radical mastectomy involves removing the entire breast, and all breast tissue extending toward the breastbone, collarbone, and to the lowest ribs; also lymph nodes in the armpit are removed and sometimes in the minor pectoral muscle.

tomical reality but simply a figurative way of referring to areas of the breast.

Quadrantectomy may be the best choice when the tumor is large or the breast is small, or both, so that removing the tumor and adequate margins requires removal of a sizable part of the breast. After surgery, the affected breast might be noticeably smaller than the healthy one. Follow-up surgery can equalize breast size and restore symmetry, either by enlarging the smaller breast or reducing the larger one.

For most early-stage breast cancers, lumpectomy includes biopsy of the lymph nodes and is nearly always followed by radiation. The combination of lumpectomy and radiation is as effective as mastectomy. This is a great blessing for women who are especially apprehensive about losing a breast.

Total Mastectomy

Total mastectomy, also called *simple mastectomy,* removes the entire breast; sometimes the nipple can be saved. No lymph nodes are removed, although a separate sentinel node biopsy, removing the first one to three axillary lymph nodes, may also be performed.

Simple mastectomy is often performed for *multifocal* breast cancers, those in which cancer is detected in more than one duct or lobe in the breast. It is also an effective *prophylactic* (preventive) procedure for women at high risk for aggressive breast cancer—those who have inherited an abnormal BRCA1 or BRCA2 gene, for example, or who have been diagnosed with lobular carcinoma *in situ* (LCIS).

Modified Radical Mastectomy

The *modified radical mastectomy,* an older approach to breast removal and rarely performed today, removes all breast tissue, covering an area from the breastbone to the back of the armpit and from the collarbone to the lower bra line, and some or all of the axillary lymph nodes. Occasionally, the small strap-like pectoralis minor muscle above the breast is removed if it interferes with node removal or if it has been invaded by cancer cells. Today, however, since the vast majority of breast cancers are discovered before they invade the chest muscles, the cancer can be removed using simpler, less invasive surgery.

The modified radical mastectomy is performed when the cancer's size, stage, or location rules out partial mastectomy. Some multifocal cancers and most stage III and stage IV cancers are treated with modified radical mastectomy because it removes not only the breast tissue but also the cancerous lymph nodes.

Sentinel Node Biopsy

Years ago, removal of the underarm lymph nodes was common with breast cancer surgery. Now, however, a simpler procedure can be performed during breast surgery to determine whether cancer has spread from the breast into nearby lymph nodes. This procedure is called a *sentinel node biopsy.* It involves sampling an underarm node called the *sentinel node,* which is usually the first node to receive lymph drainage from the breast tumor. Therefore, it is the first node in which spreading cancer cells are likely to appear.

The sentinel node biopsy is now the standard technique for testing for the spread of breast cancer into nearby lymph nodes. To perform this procedure, a surgeon first finds the sentinel node by injecting a radioactive tracer, sometimes with a blue dye, near the tumor. These substances then show up clearly on a hand-held monitor, making it possible for the surgeon to see the path the dye takes from the tumor to the lymph nodes. The first node reached by the dye and/or tracer is the sentinel node. Only if cancer is found in the sentinel node are other nodes in the area removed, because they may contain cancer cells as well.

Removing only one node or a few is a less extensive operation compared to removing all or most of the nodes. Further, the sentinel node procedure is considered as reliable as the removal of all the underarm area lymph nodes, and it is much less likely to result in complications such as lymphedema.

Postsurgical Drains

Immediately after a mastectomy or lymph node removal, the surgeon may place soft plastic tubes, or *drains,* under the skin near the closed incision. The tubes prevent discomfort and possibly infection by carrying away the tissue fluid that builds up while the incision is healing. There might be some blood in this fluid at first, but it will soon run pale yellow, collecting in a small bulb at the end of each tube. The drains are removed when the fluid diminishes, usually after five to seven days.

I had a double mastectomy and was surprised that I had very little pain. Actually, the hardest part for me was losing my hair during chemotherapy.
—Shirley, 58

Let your doctor know immediately about any severe pain, which could be a sign of *hematoma,* blood pooling in tissue at the surgical site, or internal bleeding.

Postsurgical Pain Management

Lumpectomy and mastectomy aren't generally associated with intense postoperative pain; however, managing any pain after breast surgery is essential to your comfort and to the healing process. With discomfort at a minimum, you're better able to get the rest you need to recover. Several pain management options are available during your hospital stay and during your recovery at home. Depending on your procedure, your postsurgical pain relief options while in the hospital may include pain relieving drugs, which are delivered through an intravenous line, patient-controlled analgesia (PCA), and the newer "pain relief ball." Pain relievers in pill form may also be given in the hospital or taken later at home.

Intravenous (IV) Pain Medication

A common pain management method used in hospitals following breast surgery is IV pain medication. With this method, opioid medications, such as morphine or Demerol, are delivered to you through your IV line. A nurse administers the medication at prescribed intervals, approximately every four hours. If you should continue to experience pain, notify your nurse, who may either administer another dose or consult with your surgeon about adjusting the dosage.

Patient-Controlled Analgesia (PCA)

During a hospital stay, pain relief may be administered through *patient-controlled analgesia (PCA)*. With PCA, pain medications, such as morphine, Demerol, or Dilaudid, are delivered through your intravenous line. The IV line is attached to a computerized pump that is usually mounted on a pole near your bed. When you feel pain, you simply press a button to activate the pump, which delivers a dose of medication. The pump is calibrated so that it is impossible to give yourself too many dosages.

It's usually best to give yourself small, frequent doses of the pain medication to provide steady relief. Waiting until your pain gets worse is not advisable and may make it more difficult for you to get comfortable again.

Pain Relief Ball

A newer pain management option used during a hospital stay is the ON-Q pain relief system, commonly called a *pain relief ball*. At the end of a breast operation, the surgeon inserts a small catheter into the incision site; this catheter delivers a continuous infusion of local anesthetic. The catheter is attached to a small ball, a high-tech balloon filled with anesthetic. The system infuses anesthetic directly into the surgical site for up to five days, providing ongoing pain relief. The pain relief ball reduces the incidence of breakthrough pain and reduces the need for narcotic medications, which usually cause drowsiness and decreased mental alertness.

Opioid Medications

Opioid medications, also called narcotics or opiates, are commonly taken in pill form and are used to alleviate moderate to severe pain in the days following a mastectomy or lumpectomy. However, many women find that they need the medication for only a few days, if any, following surgery.

Opioids are associated with certain side effects, including nausea, sleepiness, constipation, and slowed breathing. Opioids commonly given during a hospital stay include morphine and Demerol. Commonly prescribed opioids for use at home include Tylenol with codeine, Vicodin, Percocet, and Darvocet. Although these medications can be habit-forming, they will not lead to addiction when taken for short periods of time. The drugs can be obtained only through a physician's prescription.

Non-opioid Medications

Non-opioid pain relievers are non-narcotic, and many of them do not require a doctor's prescription. Designed to control mild to moderate pain, these medications include acetaminophen and nonsteroidal anti-inflammatory drugs (NSAIDs), such as ibuprofen and naproxen. Even though these drugs may not require a prescription, it's important to check with your doctor before taking them. Side effects are rarely associated with acetaminophen when taken for short periods. NSAIDs, however, can cause stomach pain, heartburn, dizziness, and constipation. Inform your doctor if you experience any side effects.

Recovery after Breast Surgery

Once your breast surgery is over, your recovery begins. Recovery from lumpectomy is relatively quick. However, recovery from mastectomy or mastectomy with lymph node removal requires more time, and complete recovery may take six to eight weeks. No matter which kind of surgery you've had, you'll notice improvement with each passing day.

If you've had a lumpectomy, you can expect to return to normal activities, such as walking, showering, and driving, within a day or two. Most women feel well enough to return to work within a few days. If you have had a sentinel node biopsy as part of your lumpectomy, it make take a few extra days before you're ready to return to work and other normal activities.

If you've had a mastectomy, it will be a week or more before you're ready to return to normal activities. If you've had a mastectomy with lymph node removal, you're likely to need some assistance with everyday tasks, such as washing your hair or caring for your children. Following mastectomy with or without lymph node removal, your return to work depends in part on the type of work you do.

If you have an office job, you'll be able to return to work sooner than if your work involves heavy lifting or strenuous labor. Some women return to work within a week; others take two or more weeks before going back to work.

Have someone with you before and after your surgery. My eighty-year-old mother was with me and she kept saying she felt so useless because she couldn't do any house-work or laundry for me. But she didn't realize what a help she was just by being there. It made a total difference.

—Marie, 45

Possible Side Effects of Surgery

Hematoma

A hematoma is a potential postsurgical complication that occurs when blood pools at the surgery site as a result of a leaking or ruptured blood vessel. Hematomas that occur in the breast after surgery may feel like a lump and may be painful. It is important to report this to your surgeon right away since a hematoma can cause tissue death in the area in which the bleeding occurs.

Anxiety and Depression

Some women are depressed after even the most success-ful surgery. Your body's response to the trauma of surgery can make you sad or anxious, as can the mental stress of a cancer diagnosis.

If you had a mastectomy, your first look at the place where your breast used to be may be difficult. You might even be a little afraid of seeing the surgery site after the bandages are removed. But putting it off will only create greater anxiety. When the time comes, you might want your partner or close friend there to "hold your hand."

Many women actually aren't as upset over their appearance after having had a breast removed as they expected to be. Relief that the tumor is gone usually outweighs their distress about scarring and even their very natural grief over losing a breast.

Restricted Arm Mobility and Numbness

If your lymph nodes were removed, your arm may be stiff for a few days to a few weeks. Physical therapy can help. You'll probably be shown some easy stretching and pulling exercises that will immediately improve your mobility. Eventually you'll have full, normal use of your arm. Even if small portions of muscle have been removed, your strength will return. During lymph node removal, a nerve may have been cut. This is normal and not a cause for worry, though it can cause some unpleasant symptoms. Your upper arm might be numb, and starting a few days after the operation, you may feel tingling, sharp pains, or squeezing pressure. These sensations will go away in a week or two, although in a few cases (2 to 3 percent) a chronic ache remains.

Phantom Breast

Up to 80 percent of women who have had a mastectomy report that they can "feel" the missing breast, much as people "feel" a limb that has been amputated. If your breast tumor was painful, you might feel the "ghost" of that pain for weeks or months after your surgery. Some women have "phantom breast" sensations on and off for years—not painful, simply there. These sensations are being recalled by the brain, which does not forget. They do not mean the cancer has returned. Nevertheless, it is important to check with your doctor if any new or unusual pain begins, one that has not already been identified as a phantom sensation.

Lymphedema

If your arm should become inflamed—brought on by anything from a mosquito bite to a strained muscle—your body sends extra lymph fluid, which carries infection-fighting white blood cells, to the site of the inflammation. But if the lymph nodes and vessels have been removed from that side of your body, they're no longer available to drain away excess lymph. With nowhere to go, the fluid collects in your arm, causing it to swell.

This condition, called *lymphedema,* occurs in up to 20 percent of women who have had axillary dissection. The risk of lymphedema is lowest with sentinel node biopsy and highest with complete axillary dissection.

Lymphedema is not life-threatening, but it can be painful and needs prompt treatment. If the symptoms are ignored, the fluid can become infected and, in severe cases, there can be permanent damage to the arm.

Because you can develop lymphedema anytime, even years after your surgery, you'll need to make prevention a lifelong regimen. This means maintaining a healthy weight and avoiding injury, infection, constriction, muscle strain, and temperature extremes, starting immediately after your surgery.

Call your doctor right away if you have swelling or pain in your arm; if an injury becomes puffy or tender; if your skin feels hot or is inflamed in any way—a rash, itching, or redness—or if you have a fever or flu-like symptoms. Antibiotics and diuretics, given early on, can help, as can physical therapy and specialized massages given by a lymphedema therapist.

For more information about lymphedema, contact the National Lymphedema Network, listed in the Resources section at the back of this book.

Infection

If you notice even a slight swelling of your affected arm soon after mastectomy, or if swelling, redness, or warmth occurs under the incision, it could be a sign of infection. Notify your doctor immediately. Such infections can be serious and should be treated without delay.

Postsurgical Prognosis

After your surgery, when the pathologist has examined the tumor and other tissues that were removed, your doctor will have a better idea about the need for additional treatment. The best possible news would be that the entire tumor and a clear margin have been removed, lymph node analysis shows no cancer cells, and you can expect a full recovery.

Tips for Preventing Lymphedema

- Lift nothing heavier than ten pounds with the affected arm while you're healing.

- Any exercise program or physical activity involving the arm should begin gradually and include frequent rest breaks.

- Get in the habit of consistent low-impact exercise, such as walking, swimming, or stretching.

- Don't carry a heavy purse over the affected shoulder.

- Be very protective of the affected arm to avoid injury that could lead to infection. Keep it clean. Use sunscreen and insect repellent. Use moisturizer to avoid chapping and cuticle cream to avoid hangnails (and don't cut your cuticles). Use an electric shaver, not a razor, to shave your underarms; don't use chemical hair removers. Protect your hands and arms when cooking or taking food out of a hot oven. Wear protective gloves for gardening and yard work, and rubber gloves when you're cleaning with chemicals and doing the dishes.

- Ask medical personnel not to use the affected arm to take your blood pressure, draw blood, or give an injection.

- If you get even a tiny cut or puncture, wash it with soap and water, apply an antibacterial ointment, and keep an eye on it for signs of infection.

- If you plan to take a long trip by air, consider wearing a compression garment to keep swelling down. Compression garments are sold online, in mail-order catalogs, and at many pharmacies. If you need a professionally fitted or custom-fitted compression garment, ask your doctor where you can obtain one in your area.

- Ask your doctor or a physical therapist for post-mastectomy exercises you can do to reduce the risk of lymphedema.

The majority of women with breast cancer are cured. Even so, you'll need close follow-up, since not even the best outcome can guarantee that every cancer cell is gone or that cancer will not return. Getting rid of remaining cancer after surgery is the purpose of *adjuvant therapy*—treatment given after the primary treatment (surgery, in this case) to improve the chance for a cure. Adjuvant therapy may be *local*—for example, radiation directed at the cancer site—or *systemic,* affecting the entire body, as with chemotherapy and hormone-blocking and targeted therapies.

If lymph nodes removed during surgery test positive for cancer or if your cancer was of a comparatively rare type that has a high risk of recurrence, your doctor will prescribe one or more forms of adjuvant therapy. If your tumor was node-negative (that is, with no cancer found in the lymph nodes), the doctor will probably order more tests to find out if you could benefit from adjuvant therapies as protection against recurrence.

The long-term outlook—your prognosis—depends on many factors, including your overall health, your individual anatomy, and your responses to therapy. Thus, your doctors will not be able to guarantee a particular prognosis. At best, they can tell you about general patterns of recovery, or recurrence, in cases similar to yours.

However, no two cases are exactly alike. Many women meet bad news with a positive attitude and live longer than their prognosis seemed to predict. Meanwhile, new discoveries and treatments continually emerge, lengthening lives and instantly making older statistics obsolete. Continuing developments in therapy hold great promise for breast cancer patients.

5

Breast Reconstruction

$\mathscr{I}$t has been said that mastectomy treats the disease and reconstruction heals the mind. For women with breast cancer, treating the disease is the first and by far the most important consideration. Breast reconstruction is often a close second. You may be among the many women who, though forever grateful for their recovery from breast cancer, welcome the possibility of restoring the appearance of a natural breast in place of the one that was lost.

Breast reconstruction is a safe and effective option for almost any woman who has had a breast removed. In many cases, it can be done either at the time of her original breast surgery or later—even years later. Breast cancer treatment centers offer a comprehensive team approach involving a mastectomy surgeon, a reconstructive surgeon, physicians who specialize in chemotherapy and radiation, and skilled support personnel.

Is Breast Reconstruction Right for You?

The choice is intensely personal. Many women feel strong and confident without reconstruction. Much depends on your lifestyle, profession, and personal style.

An external prosthesis is an excellent alternative for women who can't have or don't want reconstruction. Today's prostheses are lighter and less bulky than the older types, and you can start wearing a prosthesis when you have healed sufficiently, often as soon as six weeks after your mastectomy. The breast-form materials can vary from silicone gel to fiberfill.

Some types are made to fit into the pockets of post-mastectomy bras; others adhere directly to the chest.

Women who choose reconstruction, however, care about more than the way they look when fully clothed. Their breasts may be important to their sexuality, confidence, and feeling of femininity. They want to feel whole as well as look whole— they want to shower, dress, walk, reach, and bend with two breasts in place. And for some women, the mastectomy scar can be an ever-present reminder of their cancer, and reconstruction is a way to put it behind them.

Choosing a Plastic Surgeon

If you are considering breast reconstruction, make an appointment with a plastic surgeon who specializes in breast reconstruction. It is important that you feel comfortable with the surgeon and confident that you can communicate openly with him or her from the time of your first consultation to your follow-up care. Be forthright with your questions. Ask about the various reconstruction procedures available and which one he or she would advise for you. Ask to see photographs of reconstructions the plastic surgeon has performed and to be put in touch with patients who have had similar procedures. It

I kept a journal through my breast cancer experience to remember things so I could help others. The day of my surgery, I gave my journal to my friends and family who were with me in the hospital, and they wrote their thoughts. Those have been the pages I have read the most.

—Marilyn, 61

is also important that the surgeon be board-certified. Being board-certified means that a plastic surgeon has participated in a residency program in both general surgery and plastic surgery and has passed comprehensive written and oral exams. Then, board certification is granted by the American Board of Plastic Surgery (ABPS).

Plastic surgeons who have earned board certification are required to be recertified every ten years. To qualify for recertification, surgeons must receive additional training on a regular basis. This is often achieved by participating in continuing medical education. In addition, surgeons must continually meet the moral and ethical standards set by the ABPS.

The Reconstruction Plan

In a breast-reconstruction procedure, the surgeon creates a breast mound as much like the natural breast as possible. The goal of breast reconstruction is to restore symmetry or evenness to the chest wall. But if only one breast is reconstructed, no matter how realistic it is, it won't look exactly like the natural breast. Thus, many women choose to modify the natural breast with an implant, reduction, or lift, so that it more closely resembles the reconstructed breast.

Breast reconstruction should never be allowed to interfere with your number-one priority—eliminating cancer from your body. Thus, the timing and technique of your recontruction surgery will depend on the scheduling of any additional treatment, such as radiation or chemotherapy.

Immediate or Delayed Reconstruction?

Don't feel pressured to make up your mind about reconstruction before your breast surgery. As mentioned earlier, you can choose reconstruction at any time. If you know ahead of time that you will want reconstruction, you and your doctor will decide when you will have it—at the time of your breast surgery, or later. There are, however, advantages to having immediate reconstruction.

- *Financial:* It costs less to have the mastectomy and the reconstruction in the same surgery than to have the procedures at different times.

- *Emotional/Psychological:* Immediate reconstruction eliminates two sources of distress—a second surgery later on, and the experience of waking from the first surgery with no breast.

- *Personal:* Some women who would be candidates for lumpectomy with radiation therapy choose instead to have mastectomy with immediate reconstruction in order to avoid radiation.

- *Geographic:* Women in rural areas where radiation is not locally available may choose mastectomy with immediate reconstruction over lumpectomy followed by radiation.

- *Practical:* Women with jobs outside the home can minimize their time away from work by consolidating the two surgeries. Stay-at-home moms won't have to arrange child care around two operations.
- *Cosmetic:* In some cases, immediate reconstruction gives a better cosmetic result.

Not every woman is a candidate for immediate reconstruction. Radiation sometimes (but not always) makes it necessary to postpone reconstruction. Delaying the procedure might also be advised for patients with advanced breast cancer.

Women whose general health is poor or who are having emotional problems are usually better off postponing reconstruction. The best time to have reconstructive surgery is not when you are in the middle of a financial crisis, divorce, or bereavement.

Delaying reconstruction gives you time to think and become informed. The decision-making process for breast surgery alone can be overwhelming. By putting off reconstruction, you can weigh your options carefully, recover from your mastectomy, and find out whether you even want or need reconstruction.

Reconstruction Options

There are several surgical options for breast reconstruction. With every option, it is important to weigh the advantages and disadvantages of both the procedure and its outcomes. Whichever method is used, the opposite breast is usually modified for the sake of symmetry, most commonly with a breast lift and sometimes with breast reduction or breast augmentation.

Reconstruction with Implants

The most common type of reconstruction uses an implant to create a breast mound. In some cases, implant reconstruction can be performed as a single-stage procedure with an implant being placed in the breast during the mastectomy procedure. In most cases, however, implant reconstruction is a two-stage process. The first stage involves the placement of a tissue expander, which can be performed immediately during your mastectomy procedure or can be delayed until several months

Breast Implant

An implant is the most common method of breast reconstruction. Typically, a tissue expander, filled gradually with saline, is used to stretch the skin so it will accommodate the insertion of an implant.

or even years later. The second stage involves replacing the tissue expander with an implant.

There are several advantages associated with reconstruction using an implant. The procedure is considered relatively simple compared to other reconstruction methods. The surgeon almost always inserts the implant using the same incision that was used for the mastectomy, which means there are no additional resulting scars. Because the surgery is limited to the breast area, recovery is quicker than with other types of reconstruction.

This reconstruction method also has its disadvantages. Implants may feel firmer than a natural breast, and symmetry may be difficult to achieve unless the other breast is modified in some way. Also, the implant will retain its shape and firmness over the years while the natural breast ages. The difference isn't generally apparent under clothing, and products called *symmetry shapers* or *balance shapers* can be tucked into the bra to even out the appearance of the breasts.

In some instances, implant reconstruction may not be right for you. If you've had radiation therapy, your skin may not have enough elasticity to be stretched adequately to accommodate an implant. Likewise, if the skin and tissue in the breast area are considered poor quality, implant surgery may not be recommended.

Stage 1: Tissue Expansion

In most cases, the first stage of implant reconstruction is *tissue expansion,* a gradual stretching of the skin and chest muscle to create a pocket for the permanent implant. At the time of your mastectomy, or in a later procedure if you are delaying reconstruction, the surgeon places a tissue expander—a temporary balloon-like device made of elastic silicone rubber—under the skin and chest muscle. Whether a tissue expander is placed at the same time as a mastectomy or in a delayed procedure, it takes approximately one to two hours. In a delayed procedure, tissue expander placement is performed using anesthesia in an operating room. The procedure may be performed on an outpatient basis, or it may require a brief hospital stay.

Approximately once every one to two weeks for two to four months, fluid is injected through a port, or entry site, that is part of the tissue expander itself or connected to a tube just under the skin. Gradually, the volume of fluid grows, the skin and muscle expand, and the pocket is created.

If you are scheduled for radiation and you are planning to undergo tissue expansion, it's recommended to have tissue expansion performed prior to beginning radiation treatments. That's because, as mentioned above, radiated skin loses its elasticity and is unable to be stretched. Once you've completed radiation treatment, your surgeon will evaluate the skin in your breast area to determine if you're a candidate for implant placement. If not, having undergone tissue expansion can still be beneficial; it can give the surgeon greater latitude in shaping your new breast using other types of reconstruction.

I was able to get through my reconstruction by telling myself, "You can do this. You're going to look great when it's over!"

—Joan, 47

During tissue expansion, you may notice some discomfort for a day or so after each injection; what you're feeling is the muscle stretching to accommodate the additional fluid. Your surgeon can prescribe pain medication if necessary, but many women alleviate any discomfort with over-the-counter medications.

Stage 2: Implant Placement

Whether an implant is placed at the same time as a mastectomy or following tissue expansion, it takes approximately one to two hours. Implant placement following tissue expansion can be performed using anesthesia on an outpatient basis, or it may require a hospital stay of one to two days. During the procedure, your doctor will remove the tissue expander, insert the permanent implant, and modify (lift, augment, or reduce) the opposite breast for symmetry or evenness.

For breast reconstruction, implants are almost always placed submuscularly, under the pectoral muscle. It's possible for an implant to be placed above the muscle, but since there is no breast tissue to cover it, the implant may be easy to feel and may not appear natural-looking. Submuscular placement generally provides a more natural look and feel.

Types of Implants

The implants used in reconstruction consist of a silicone shell and are filled with either saline or silicone gel. Saline implants are filled with sterile saline, a saltwater solution similar to the body's own fluids. If a saline implant leaks or ruptures, the saline is absorbed by the body and eliminated through urination.

Silicone gel is denser than saline, and many surgeons and women believe that silicone implants look and feel more natural than saline implants. Leaks in silicone implants aren't easy to detect, and the gel remains in the body. Controversy about silicone gel led the Food and Drug Administration (FDA) in 1992 to issue regulations on silicone-gel breast implants. The FDA didn't ban these implants—no studies have shown that they are harmful—but their use was restricted to women with breast cancer, breast injuries, or breast deformities. However, in 2006, this ban was lifted.

Silicone gel and saline implants come in a variety of shapes and textures. Implants are either round or anatomical, also called teardrop, contoured, or shaped.

- Round implants: these implants typically produce greater fullness on the top of the breast than a natural breast.

- Anatomical implants: these implants are designed to mimic the natural slope of the breast and are fuller at the bottom than at the top. Because of this, anatomical implants are often chosen for reconstruction.

An implant's outer shell can be either smooth or textured (similar to fine sandpaper). Round implants come in both varieties. Anatomical implants are available exclusively with textured shells.

Potential Complications with Implants

There are possible complications associated with breast implants. They include the following:

- scar tissue, called a *capsular contracture,* developing around the implant, causing it to be unusually firm
- infection, which may require removal of the implant or the tissue expander
- leakage, which is not hazardous but does require replacement of the implant
- extrusion, in which the skin erodes and the implant shows through. This will require surgery.

Reconstruction with Your Own Tissues
TRAM Flap Reconstruction

Breast reconstruction with your own body tissue often uses skin, fat, and muscle from the lower abdomen—a *transverse rectus abdominis myocutaneous flap,* or *TRAM flap.* In a TRAM flap procedure, blood flow to the transferred tissues is continuous. By contrast, grafted tissue is disconnected from its blood supply and quickly moved to its destination elsewhere on the body, where new blood vessels grow into it. Because all body tissues must have a blood supply to survive, any interruption in that supply can endanger the tissues.

During a TRAM flap procedure using abdominal skin, fat, and muscle, the surgeon creates a tunnel under the skin through which the tissues will be moved. They remain connected to their blood supply through a muscle that runs from the chest to the pelvis. After the muscle of the abdominal wall has been moved, mesh may be used to reinforce the abdominal wall.

71

This woman had a mastectomy at age forty-three.

This fifty-year-old woman's breast cancer in her left breast was detected early. She had a lumpectomy, in which the cancerous growth and surrounding tissue were removed.

At age forty-seven, this woman had both breasts removed. She chose a bilateral (both sides) TRAM flap reconstruction, followed by reconstruction of the nipple and areola.

This woman was forty-three-years old when diagnosed with breast cancer in her left breast. She underwent a lumpectomy, which was followed by radiation therapy. Her scar, on the right side of her left breast, is barely visible.

At age fifty, this woman had a bilateral mastectomy. She chose to have saline implants and is not planning to have nipple and areola reconstruction.

This woman, age thirty-eight at the time of her surgery, had both breasts removed. She chose to have tissue expanders with saline implants. During a second procedure, she had nipple and areola reconstruction.

At age forty-nine, this woman chose to have a lumpectomy performed on her right breast. She also underwent six weeks of radiation therapy.

Tissue expanders were inserted immediately following this forty-six-year-old woman's double mastectomy. Saline implants were placed six weeks later, followed by reconstruction of the nipple and areola.

TRAM Flap

During a TRAM flap procedure, skin, fat, and muscle from the lower abdomen is used. The rectus muscle is disconnected, but left anchored to the rib cage. Then, the skin and fat, which remain attached to the muscle, are rotated upward to form the breast. The fat tissue in the flap helps form the new breast.

At the chest site, the surgeon shapes the flap to resemble the opposite breast as closely as possible. Because abdominal fat and breast fat are about the same consistency, the new breast usually looks and feels natural. As a bonus, the patient gets a flatter abdomen, since the tissues removed are similar to those removed during a "tummy tuck."

TRAM flap surgery is more extensive than implant surgery, requiring about three to five hours for the procedure, a hospital stay of two to four days, and eight to twelve weeks for full recovery. While you are in the hospital, opioid pain medication is likely to be administered. Your surgeon will probably prescribe opioid pain medication for an additional one to two weeks at home.

If you are a good candidate for this surgery and if your plastic surgeon is well qualified and experienced with TRAM flap breast reconstruction, it is a safe procedure. Although the complication rate is low, there is the potential for infection and complete or partial loss of the transferred tissue. In addition, because the muscle of the abdominal wall has been moved up to the breast, the abdomen may be weakened, resulting in possible hernias.

Having a TRAM flap reconstruction might not be an option for you if:

- you are obese or very thin
- you have abdominal scars from previous surgery
- you are a smoker

- you have diabetes or other blood-vessel disease
- you have lung or heart disease

Free DIEP Flap Reconstruction

A newer variation of the TRAM flap is called a *DIEP (Deep Inferior Epigastric Perferater) flap.* In this procedure, skin and fat are taken from the abdomen and transferred to the breast site. No muscle is transferred, however, which eliminates the need for a mesh on the abdominal wall and lessens the risk of hernias. To create blood flow, tiny blood vessels in the transferred tissue are attached to blood vessels in the breast area. This procedure is technically challenging and requires a surgeon who is skilled in microvascular surgery.

A DIEP procedure takes approximately three to six hours and requires a hospital stay of approximately two to four days. In the hospital, opioid medications are commonly administered, and you can expect to continue taking prescribed opioid medications for one to two weeks. Full recovery takes about eight to twelve weeks. Another variation of this procedure is called the SIEA (Superficial Inferior Epigastric Artery) flap, but it is rarely used.

Latissimus Dorsi Flap Reconstruction

This procedure uses tissues from one of the *latissimus dorsi*—the broad, flat, triangular muscles on the back that are known as "lats." Skin, muscle, and fat are transferred to the front in order to re-create the breast, usually but not always in conjunction with an implant. During the procedure, which takes about two hours, a football-shaped section of skin approximately eight centimeters wide by fifteen centimeters (about three to six inches) long is tunneled under the armpit to the breast area. An implant or a tissue expander is placed in the same procedure. The main disadvantages of this reconstruction method are a scar on your back and the loss of your lat muscle. Most women, however, function just fine without it.

You can expect to spend about two days in the hospital following this procedure. Opioid pain medications are typically administered in the hospital and are often prescribed for one to two weeks during recovery at home. You can usually drive within about ten days, with full recovery expected at about eight weeks.

Latissimus Dorsi Flap Reconstruction

In this procedure, the latissimus dorsi muscle in the back is disconnected, but stays attached at the armpit. The skin and fat, attached to the muscle, are pulled around to form the breast. This procedure usually also requires an implant.

Gluteal Flap Reconstruction

Another reconstruction method uses flaps taken from the gluteal area called *SGAP (Superior Gluteal Artery Perforator)* or *IGAP (Inferior Gluteal Artery Perforator)*. This method uses skin, fat, and muscle from the upper portion of the buttock (SGAP) or lower portion of the buttock (IGAP). In this procedure, a wedge from one of the buttocks is transferred and shaped to form the new breast. The procedure is longer and more complicated than a latissimus flap or TRAM flap. The surgeon must disconnect the blood vessels and then reattach them to the chest wall using an operating microscope. The blood vessels in the buttocks are short and can only be attached to certain vessels that are difficult to reach in the chest area. Because of this, the surgery is technically challenging and not commonly performed.

This procedure is usually not recommended unless you aren't eligible for any other type of reconstruction. With this method, there's a greater risk for tissue loss, and you're left with a scar either on the upper buttock or in the crease below the buttock. Because of the nature of this surgery, lung deflation during the procedure is a risk; this can be quickly corrected should it occur.

The surgery takes approximately four to six hours and requires a hospital stay of about two days. Opioid pain relievers are generally used while in the hospital. At home, you may need to continue taking prescribed opioids for one to two weeks.

Postsurgical Pain Management

Breast reconstruction is generally associated with more pain than one might experience with lumpectomy or mastectomy, but any discomfort you may feel can be alleviated with medication. The same pain management options used following a mastectomy are used to minimize postoperative pain after breast reconstruction. These options include opioids—which may be administered intravenously, through a "pain pump," with a pain relief ball, or in pill form.

During implant reconstruction, I was uncomfortable sleeping on my stomach and on my side. I learned to prop up pillows at my back and under my arm to sleep more comfortably.

—Suzanne, 58

If you're like most women and require a brief hospital stay following breast reconstruction, opioid pain relievers are likely to be administered during this time. Doctors also commonly prescribe opioids for an additional one to two weeks once you return home. You may switch to over-the-counter, non-opioid pain relievers as soon as you feel ready.

Talk to your surgeon prior to your surgery about how your pain will be managed. It's important to have this matter clarified before you enter the operating room.

Recovery after Breast Reconstruction

In most cases, you can expect your recovery from breast reconstruction to take more time than your recovery from a mastectomy. In general, recovering from breast reconstruction that involves tissues from other areas of the body takes more time than reconstruction using implants. Depending on the type of reconstruction you have, your return to normal activities, such as driving and walking, may take one to two weeks, and, in some cases, even longer. Full recovery from breast reconstruction can take as little as five weeks or as much as twelve weeks and depends largely on the type of surgery you choose.

Nipple-Areola Reconstruction

Nipple-areola reconstruction can be performed once you've fully recovered from your implant or flap procedure. The nipple is formed from tissue on the newly reconstructed breast. The areola around the nipple can be re-created by grafting a small piece of skin from elsewhere on the body. This skin graft is usually taken from the abdomen, but can also come from the upper inner thigh or the gluteal crease. After the newly formed nipple and areola have healed, the surgeon can tattoo the areola to make it darker and more natural looking; this can be performed, with a local anesthetic, during an office visit. If you prefer, you can eliminate the areola skin graft and simply have an areola tattooed on the breast mound, but this isn't as natural-looking as a grafted areola.

Nipple-areola reconstruction takes about one hour and is performed on an outpatient basis using anesthesia or a local anesthetic. Recovery time is minimal. Because it contributes to the natural look of the breast, the majority of women who choose breast reconstruction also opt for nipple-areola reconstruction.

Insurance Coverage

Since passage of the 1998 *Women's Health and Cancer Rights Act,* insurance companies have been required by law to pay for reconstruction of a surgically treated breast and for surgery on the opposite breast if needed. Physical therapy to restore full arm movement after mastectomy, with or without reconstruction, may also be covered by insurance.

Breast Forms or Prostheses

If you decide not to have reconstruction, you can always wear a prosthesis. Many women forgo prostheses as well as reconstruction, for any of a number of reasons: They feel no

Breast forms are made with silicone gel. *Photo courtesy of Amoena.*

need to conceal the fact that they've had breast surgery, or they're small-breasted to start with, or they like to wear loose clothing, or they just don't want to be bothered with finding, fitting, and wearing an artificial breast.

It's your call. There are as many ways for a woman to feel and look comfortable and confident as there are women.

If you're at your best in tailored, well-fitting clothes, there is no need to sacrifice the look you want. Your surgeon or hospital can put you in touch with a volunteer who is knowledgeable about the numerous and attractive styles of breast prostheses. Some are quite economical and look as good as the pricey ones. The cost can vary widely and is often covered by insurance.

Today's breast forms are not only more convenient and comfortable than older ones but can also be matched to your other breast in size, weight, and appearance. Some attach to the chest wall with the help of a small piece of Velcro-like fabric that can remain painlessly in place for several days or weeks. Others can be secured inside a bra. There are special prostheses for swimming or sports, as well as swimsuits and other garments designed for women who have had mastectomies.

You'll find breast prostheses in catalogs, on the Internet, or in specialized lingerie shops, where you can be fitted for one that is precisely the right size and shape for you.

6

Radiation Therapy

*R*adiation therapy is often prescribed as a follow-up treatment to surgery for breast cancer. Statistics show that radiation therapy can substantially reduce the risk of local recurrence. Cells that are damaged by radiation therapy lose their ability to reproduce, making radiation effective against fast-growing cancer cells. Healthy tissues may also be damaged during treatment; however, the healthy cells heal while the cancer cells do not. Radiation therapy is usually quite tolerable for most women.

Choosing a Radiation Oncologist

A *radiation oncologist* is a physician who specializes in radiation therapy for cancer patients. Most likely, your surgeon or another physician will refer you to this specialist. The initial consultation is an opportunity for you to discuss treatment benefits and risks with the radiation oncologist, who in all likelihood is someone your referring doctor has worked with many times. You are under no obligation to choose this oncologist, and it is your prerogative to ask for another referral.

Consider having a friend or partner go with you to at least the first meeting with the radiation oncologist—to take notes or ask questions you might forget to ask. Write down as many questions as you can think of in advance. Here are examples of the kinds of things you'll probably be wondering about:

- Will radiation improve my prognosis? To what extent?
- How many treatments will I need? How often will they be given, and for how long?

- Which area will be targeted?
- How much healthy tissue will be exposed to radiation, and where?
- What side effects should I expect, and how can I manage them?

If you live in a rural area or small town, find out where the nearest qualified radiation facility is located. Ask your surgeon or contact the Cancer Information Service of the National Cancer Institute (*see* the Resources section at the back of this book).

Don't rule out radiation if you live too far from a radiation facility to commute every day. If you don't have friends or relatives who live near a facility and can offer you a place to stay, and you can't afford to stay six weeks or more in a hotel, contact the radiation facility's social worker or patient-support representative. Many medical centers employ people whose job it is to help out with everything from lodging and transportation to financial and family counseling. Programs such as the American Cancer Society's Hope Lodges provide not only free temporary housing during cancer treatment but also a supportive, homelike environment.

Finally, a diagnostic test, described in chapter 2, may also be helpful in determining whether you would benefit from radiation therapy (or chemotherapy). You may recall, the Oncotype DX test examines the activity of twenty-one genes and indicates whether the cancer is likely to recur. You would be a candidate for an Oncotype DX text if:

- you've recently been diagnosed with stage I or II invasive breast cancer
- the cancer is estrogen-receptor-positive
- there is no cancer in your lymph nodes (lymph node-negative breast cancer)
- you and your doctor are making decisions about radiation (or chemotherapy)

Talk to your physician if any of these factors apply to you.

When Is Radiation Used?

After Lumpectomy

Radiation therapy after lumpectomy destroys random cancer cells that might remain in the breast or lymph nodes even when the entire tumor, a clean margin, and any of the lymph nodes have been removed. With external beam radiation, the entire breast area is treated by radiation after lumpectomy, including the site from which the tumor was removed.

After Mastectomy

When the entire breast has been removed and no remaining cancer is detected, radiation is usually unnecessary. If the tumor was large, however, or if cancer was found in the margins or in several lymph nodes, radiation is advisable as a safeguard in case surgery did not remove all the cancer cells.

Similarly, if a large amount of cancer has been removed from the inner breast (near the breastbone) or has been found in several underarm nodes, radiation may be used on the lymph nodes behind the breastbone and above the collarbone, since these lymph nodes might also contain cancer cells.

Finally, when a large tumor, five centimeters (two inches) or more, has been shrunk by chemotherapy or hormone-blocking therapy before surgery, radiation after the surgery can reduce the risk of local recurrence.

Delivery of Radiation Therapy

Radiation therapy may be delivered in one of two ways. First, the standard form of radiation therapy involves delivery of radiation externally—called *external beam radiation*. This form of treatment may be used after mastectomy; it can also be used after a lumpectomy.

The second approach, which may be used after a lumpectomy, is referred to as *brachytherapy*. This form of radiation is delivered internally to the lumpectomy cavity through tiny tubes that are inserted into the breast.

External Beam Radiation

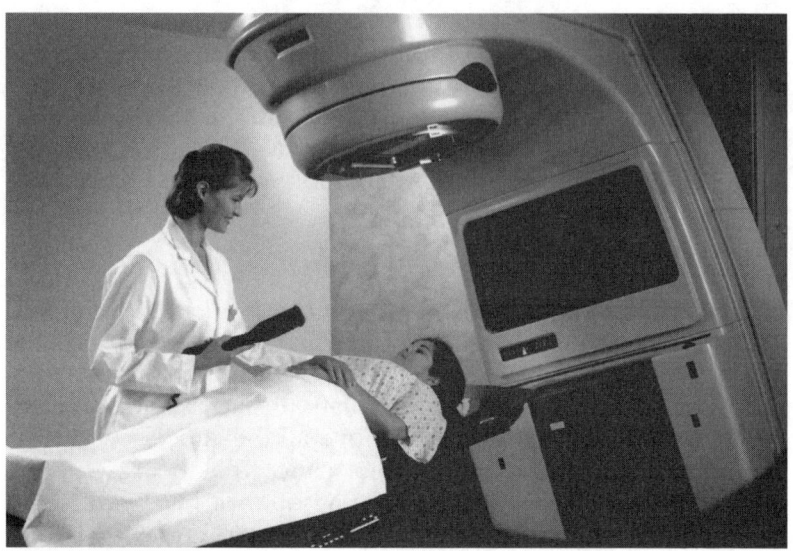

A patient receiving an external beam radiation treatment. *Photo courtesy of Siemen's Medical Systems, Inc.*

Simulation Appointment

If you are to receive external beam radiation, you'll have what's called a simulation appointment with your radiation oncologist and his or her team prior to your first treatment. This is a planning session during which the team will determine the precise area to receive the radiation treatment. This plan will be followed carefully during each treatment.

During the simulation, a customized mold will be made for your arm, back, and neck. This mold will be used during your treatments to hold your upper body in place.

Part of the simulation appointment will also involve the application of some tiny tattoos—black dots about the size of a pinhead—on your chest to indicate the area to be treated. Most women do not find these tattoos to be cosmetically bothersome; however, they can be removed professionally with a laser.

Once the simulation is completed, you'll be scheduled for your first radiation treatment.

External Beam Radiation Therapy

External radiation for cancer treatment reaches its target in the form of a radiation beam, delivered by a machine called a *linear accelerator.* The treatments are painless, much like having an X-ray.

External beam radiation treatments, including preparation, last about ten minutes. A typical treatment schedule is Monday through Friday for three and a half to seven weeks. You're asked not to wear deodorants, powders, creams, lotions, or fragrances when you go to the treatment center. Upon arriving, you'll remove your clothes from the waist up and change into a gown. You'll soon become familiar with the treatment routine.

Radiation was not a bad experience. I actually came to enjoy going every day. In fact, I cried on my last visit because everyone there was so wonderful to me.
—Sandy, 44

A specially trained radiation therapist will deliver your treatments. For an external beam radiation treatment, the therapist will usually have you lie on your back; however, some women receive the treatment lying on their abdomen. You'll be asked to lie perfectly still. The radiation machine, which will be above you, will deliver radiation to the tattooed area. The machine will be rotated above you and carefully positioned in two or more places during a treatment session.

Accelerated Breast Radiation Therapy

Some treatment centers are working to shorten the length of time during which whole breast, external beam radiation therapy is given. For example, some doctors are delivering higher doses of radiation over a span of three weeks instead of the typical period of several weeks. This accelerated approach is called *hypofractionated radiation therapy.*

Boost Treatments

Your initial radiation therapy might be followed immediately by boost treatments that zero in on the site from which the tumor was removed. Whether you receive this "boost" dose of radiation will depend on factors such as age, the size and type of your tumor, the width of the margins, and the size of your breast.

Studies show that boost treatments further reduce the risk of recurrence for all women; however, not every woman will need them. Boost treatments may use external beam therapy, or the radiation may be delivered internally with brachytherapy.

External Boost Treatments

The external boost treatments are similar to the standard external beam treatments; however, the area being treated will be smaller. These boost treatments are usually given daily for one week.

Internal Boost Treatments

The internal boost treatments with brachytherapy may be an option for a woman who has had a lumpectomy. The radiation is delivered to the tumor site from inside the body. Brachytherapy begins with the surgical insertion of multiple tiny catheters into the area from which the tumor was surgically removed. Then, during a treatment, a radioactive seed is delivered into each catheter.

The brachytherapy may be given at a "high-dose rate" or "low-dose rate." The difference between the two doses relates to the time it takes to complete the treatments. The high-dose-rate brachytherapy is given on an outpatient basis, twice a day for two to three days; each treatment usually lasts a few minutes. The low-dose brachytherapy is given continuously over a two-day period on an inpatient basis.

Once the treatment is completed, the tiny tubes are removed. If you must travel to a radiation facility for treatment, brachytherapy reduces travel time.

Accelerated Partial Breast Irradiation

A newer form of treatment, *accelerated partial breast irradiation (APBI),* is becoming an increasingly popular form of radiation treatment for women who have had lumpectomies. APBI can be delivered with external beam radiation or with brachytherapy. It delivers radiation to only part of the breast rather than the whole breast. As a result, the treatment minimizes radiation exposure to healthy tissue, and the treatment takes only about five days rather than several weeks. It can also be delivered prior to chemotherapy. Most women report few side effects.

Who is a candidate for partial breast irradiation? Generally, good candidates are women with smaller tumors who have clear surgical margins, have only one site of disease, and have minimal lymph node involvement.

Is APBI effective? Yes it is, according to a 2009 study done at the William Beaumont Hospital in Michigan. This study, which followed up with women ten years after their treatments, showed the same low rate of recurrence (5 percent) among women who received whole breast radiation and those who received partial breast radiation.

Radiation Therapy Side Effects

Because radiation is a localized treatment, it typically has only localized side effects. The majority of women go through radiation treatment with few or minimal side effects. The potential temporary side effects of radiation include:

- swelling of the area
- skin redness, resembling a sunburn
- aches and pains in the treated area (This is not a sign of cancer recurring.)
- fatigue

There is the potential for long-term side effects after radiation therapy. These may include:

- reduced skin elasticity
- a breast that is firmer than normal
- puffiness or change in the size of the treated breast
- change in sensitivity to touch or pressure
- slight darkening or thickening of the skin
- chronic twinges or slight aching in the breast
- arm lymphedema (if lymph nodes received radiation)

Other complications are not likely, but are possible. *Radiation pneumonitis* is a lung reaction that may occur during treatment or weeks to months after treatment; it causes fever, coughing, and shortness of breath. It usually does not require treatment and goes away in a few weeks. It is also possible for radiation therapy to damage the heart; however, modern treatments strive to avoid this. Women who smoke or who have pre-existing heart disease may be more at risk. Finally, women under age forty-five have a slight risk (1 in 1,000) for developing cancer five to twenty years later; such cancer may develop in the skin, muscle, bone, or lung.

Radiation therapy for breast cancer will not affect your fertility, menstrual periods, or reproductive system. Some women can breast-feed with the untreated breast and sometimes with the treated breast.

Take especially good care of yourself during your radiation treatment period. These self-care basics can ease your side effects and keep you more comfortable:

- Get plenty of rest.
- Use lukewarm water and mild soap to cleanse the treated area. Do not scrub.
- Wear loose, comfortable clothing during the weeks of treatment. If possible, don't wear a bra.
- Don't use powders, creams, lotions, or deodorants on the treated area before a treatment.
- Ask your radiation oncologist to recommend a cream to use on treated skin after treatments.
- Shield the treated area from sunlight. Some physicians recommend wearing protective clothing or using sun-screen for up to a year following radiation treatment.
- Don't try to scrub or rub off the ink marks—they will fade in time. Tattoos, however, are permanent.

These measures may help keep you comfortable, lift your spirits, manage your side effects, and help you feel more in control during this time of healing.

7

Systemic Therapies

*A*fter breast cancer surgery, it's possible that some cancer cells still remain in the body. Therefore, *systemic therapy* is recommended to increase long-term survival. This form of treatment uses drugs that travel through the bloodstream to fight cancer. One of the systemic treatments you may be most familiar with is *chemotherapy,* which works to destroy undetected cancer cells that may have spread to areas beyond the location of the original tumor. When chemotherapy follows a primary treatment, such as surgery, the follow-up treatment is called an *adjuvant therapy.*

Another systemic treatment, *hormone-blocking therapy,* works much differently than chemotherapy. Rather than destroy cancer cells, hormone-blocking drugs keep them from reproducing. They do this by depriving cancer cells of the hormones they depend upon.

Yet another form of systemic treatment, *targeted therapy,* involves using drugs to defend against cancer by attaching to specific molecules within or on the surface of cells. As the medical community has learned more about the gene changes in cells that cause cancer, they have been able to develop drugs that target these changes.

Your Medical Oncologist

Adjuvant therapies, such as chemotherapy, are administered by a *medical oncologist,* a physician who specializes in systemic cancer treatments. Your surgeon will refer you to a well-qualified medical oncologist in your area. This physician

Chemotherapy Treatment

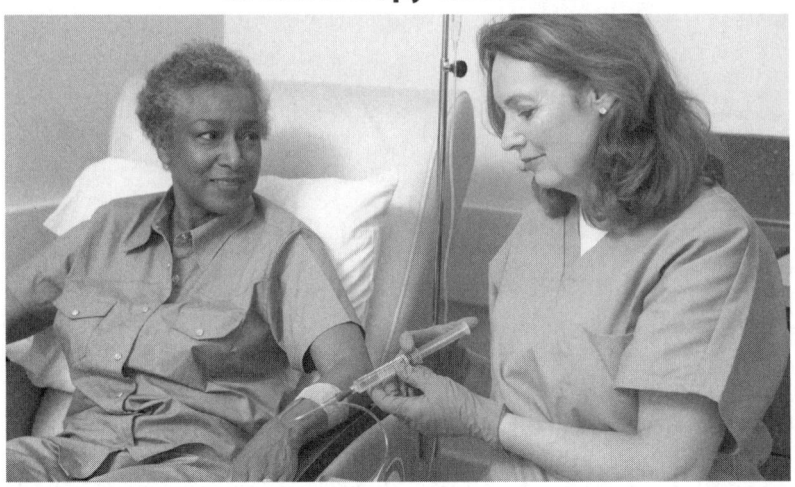

Most chemotherapy treatments are delivered intravenously. Treatments are usually given after surgery, but are sometimes given to shrink a tumor prior to surgery.

should be board-certified in medical oncology. To be board-certified, a doctor must have the prescribed training and pass rigorous examinations. This specialist should be someone who inspires your confidence, listens carefully to your questions and concerns, and puts you at ease. You may find it helpful to arrive at each appointment with a list of your questions.

It is important for your doctor to know what medications you are taking, including prescription drugs, vitamins, herbs, and over-the-counter drugs such as aspirin, ibuprofen, sleep aids, and cold medicines.

Chemotherapy

The decision to use chemotherapy depends on such factors as the type of tumor, how aggressive it is, and a patient's age and overall health. Chemotherapy is usually recommended when cancer has spread from the breast to the underarm lymph nodes or when a tumor has aggressive characteristics, whether the nodes are cancerous or not. With smaller tumors and no evidence of cancer in the nodes, chemotherapy is prescribed only on a case-by-case basis.

The term *chemotherapy* refers to a group of drugs, just as the term *antibiotic* refers to many different medications. Chemotherapy drugs act against all rapidly dividing cells—not only cancer cells but also hair cells, gastrointestinal cells, and bone-marrow cells. This explains why hair often falls out during chemotherapy.

The chemotherapy agents listed below each behave differently against cancer cells. Doctors prescribe them in combinations that maximize their benefits. The most commonly used chemotherapy regimens include:

- docetaxel and cyclophosphamide
- adriamycin and cyclophosphamide, which are often followed by docetaxel or paclitaxel (with or without trastuzumab)
- carboplatin, docetaxel, and trastuzumab
- cyclophosphamide with methotrexate and 5-fluoro-uracil
- carboplatinum or cisplatinum

Other chemotherapy drug combinations may also be utilized; these regimens change frequently as new drugs become available.

Chemotherapy Treatments

There are chemotherapy drugs that you can take at home in pill, capsule, or liquid form. More often, however, chemotherapy drugs are injected or infused (slowly dripped) directly into a vein; occasionally, the chemotherapy is injected into a muscle, under the skin, or into the cancer itself. Only someone thoroughly trained and experienced in the use of chemotherapy can administer drugs in this way, so each treatment requires a visit to the oncologist's office.

After surgery and chemotherapy, I also had radiation. I got great support from family and friends. I kept telling myself I would beat this disease.

—Shirley, 58

Chemotherapy may be given in a vein, or through a small port into the vein that is surgically implanted just under the skin. The port is attached to a tube leading directly to a large vein, and it remains in place until all chemotherapy treatments are finished.

Chemotherapy as Treatment for Breast Cancer

Chemotherapy has been used to treat breast cancer since the late 1960s. However, it was during the 1970s that its curative powers became known. During this time, chemotherapy was determined to be an effective treatment for women whose breast cancers had spread to nearby lymph nodes. The medical community also learned chemotherapy dramatically decreased a woman's rate of breast cancer recurrence. The increase in the survival rate was striking, and by the 1990s, chemotherapy was recommended for women with stages I through III breast cancer.

The port has numerous advantages. It's usually more convenient for patients since it eliminates the need for repeated needle "sticks." A port is also useful for the delivery of certain medications or when an infusion over several days is needed. It's also useful when conditions such as swelling or obesity make it difficult for medical professionals to find a vein.

If you receive chemotherapy, the dose will be customized especially for you. The goal is to kill as many cancer cells as possible without putting you at undue risk. The range of acceptable dosages is small, but within that range, there is room for differences of opinion. Some oncologists prefer to give the highest acceptable dosages less often; others prefer to give lower dosages more often. As a consequence, your treatments might be weekly, every other week, or even monthly. The nature of each drug and drug combination also determines how often it is given.

Timing of Chemotherapy Cycles

The earlier chemotherapy is given after surgery, the better; there will be fewer cancer cells to attack and the likelihood of success is enhanced. A common chemotherapy regimen begins two to four weeks after surgery and continues for three months to six months.

There is a reason why chemotherapy is given in cycles, or "waves." This approach kills more cancer cells. The first wave of treatment will kill many cells that are just then in the process of dividing. It will miss cells that are at rest, but will kill some of these in the next wave. The cycles of treatment continue with the intent of destroying as many remaining cancer cells as possible. The number and duration of cycles depend on the drugs being used, their dosages, and the stage of the cancer.

Most chemotherapy is given after surgery; however, in some cases, it is better to give the chemotherapy prior to surgery. This approach is called *neoadjuvant chemotherapy.* The intent of this therapy is to shrink a tumor prior to surgical removal. This form of chemotherapy is always recommended for inflammatory breast cancer and often for larger breast cancers; it is especially recommended if a woman is interested in shrinking a tumor so that she can undergo a lumpectomy, which will preserve her breast.

Side Effects of Chemotherapy

Despite the amazing advances in chemotherapy over the years, you'll probably feel a little nervous at first about side effects. It might help to remember that these are only temporary. Side effects vary widely from person to person and drug to drug. Not everyone will have problems with nausea and hair loss. You might be on a different chemotherapy regimen and schedule; you might react differently to the drugs being used; and you might be given different medications to control your side effects.

> *I had two rounds of chemotherapy and radiation. But every day puts you in a better place. The greatest lesson I learned was that hard times don't last. You will feel better. Things will get better.*
> —*Ann, 53*

Low Blood Count

At every treatment, you'll probably have blood drawn and tested. Your doctor will want to make sure that you have adequate levels of red blood cells, white blood cells, and platelets, all of which are essential to your health. All three of these blood components are produced in the *bone marrow,* and when chemotherapy damages bone-marrow cells, the cell-production process slows down. This affects the body in a different way for each component.

Red blood cells carry the oxygen that gives the body fuel for energy, so a reduction in red blood cells causes fatigue and sometimes shortness of breath.

White blood cells fight infection, and when there are fewer white blood cells, the risk of infection increases. If your white blood cell count gets dangerously low, your doctor might briefly postpone your chemotherapy treatment or lower your dosage. Alternatively, he or she might recommend an injection of a growth factor that causes bone marrow to produce and release more white blood cells, enabling you to remain on your normal chemotherapy dosage and schedule. Even so, you will be particularly vulnerable to infection during periods when your cell counts are low, so any signs of infection, such as fever, redness, pain, or swelling, should be promptly reported to your medical oncologist.

When the level of *blood platelets*—cells that aid clotting—becomes low, you may have nosebleeds or bleeding gums, bruise easily, or bleed longer after cutting yourself. If any of these symptoms occurs, notify your doctor right away.

Nausea

Nausea has not been completely eliminated as a side effect of chemotherapy. However, fewer and fewer patients experience nausea during chemotherapy, and those who do can usually manage it well with over-the-counter medicines or prescription drugs, either taken orally or injected. The drugs used most often for nausea are Zofran, Compazine, and Phenergan. If nausea is severe, the drug Emend, taken orally an hour before treatment, is very beneficial. Patients who do experience nausea say it usually lasts a day or two and then subsides.

Eating slowly, and eating small amounts of food at a time—especially dry foods such as toast or crackers—may help, whereas eating heavily right before a treatment is not advised.

Joint Pain

After chemotherapy, about 5 percent of patients notice short-term or lasting joint pain. Most physicians recommend over-the-counter anti-inflammatory drugs such as ibuprofen. Some doctors say their patients report success in relieving joint pain with chondroitin and glucosamine, nonprescription supplements available at most pharmacies and health-food stores.

Hair Loss

Losing hair is one of the side effects that women find especially emotionally painful. However, the hair not only grows back, but it's not uncommon for the new hair to be thicker, curlier, or even a slightly different color. In some women, the hair only gets thinner rather than falls out completely. Hair loss or thinning can start a few days after chemotherapy begins, but two or three weeks later is more usual.

I didn't want to go through chemo; I didn't want to lose my hair, but I did. Later, at stop signs, I used to whip off my wig on the hot drives home from work and enjoy the astonishment on the faces of other drivers.

—Suzanne, 58

If you do lose your hair—including eyebrows, lashes, and body hair—it will probably grow back completely within three to five months after you complete chemotherapy. Regrowth sometimes starts even before chemotherapy has ended.

Before your treatment begins, you might want to buy an attractive hairpiece that matches your hair color and is cut and styled the way you like it, or stock up on hats, scarves, and turbans if you find wigs too uncomfortable. Being prepared will help you manage hair loss if it does occur.

A program called "Look Good...Feel Better" puts cancer patients in touch with cosmetologists who provide free advice on makeup and wigs. For more information, see the American Cancer Society listing in the Resources section at the back of this book.

Memory Loss

Some women having chemotherapy report a condition they occasionally refer to as "chemo brain"—a faulty memory that may not improve after the treatments have ended. These women say they are forgetful or "fuzzy-headed" and find it harder to concentrate than they used to, though the condition is almost always mild and doesn't interfere with their ability to hold a job or go about their daily activities.

Study results haven't been unanimous on the cause of this memory loss. Some researchers believe that the problem is a direct result of chemotherapy, most often associated with drugs in the taxane class. Others claim that the memory problems have more to do with hormonal changes, the trauma of being diagnosed with and treated for breast cancer, and sleep disruption.

Fatigue

Women who experience fatigue during the course of their chemotherapy treatments say the first day after treatment is often the most difficult, but the fatigue often lessens in subsequent days. A flexible schedule helps. If you find yourself tired late in the day, try making time for a nap before dinner.

> *I thought if there's a chance chemotherapy will kill any cancer left in my body, the six-month inconvenience was worth it.*
> *—Dianna, 44*

Fatigue may increase as the months of chemotherapy progress, and it may persist for a year or two after treatment ends. In cases where fatigue is caused by low blood counts, drugs that stimulate production of red or white blood cells can help. Two such drugs are *epoetin alfa* (Procrit), which is a synthetic form of the human protein *erythropoietin,* and *filgrastim* (Neupogen).

Menopausal Symptoms

Some women stop menstruating during chemotherapy and also may experience the night sweats and hot flashes common in menopause. Other menopausal symptoms include vaginal dryness, fatigue, depression, insomnia, and weight gain.

Younger women usually begin menstruating again after chemotherapy, but women in or near their forties may not. For those who do resume menstruating, fertility is not thought to be affected; they can still conceive and bear children. Remember, temporary cessation of menses during chemotherapy does not necessarily mean you are infertile. So use appropriate birth control measures to prevent pregnancy since chemotherapy drugs can cause birth defects.

Other Side Effects

Other side effects can include mouth sores and taste changes, poor appetite, diarrhea or constipation, tingling or numbness, irritated skin, fluid retention, and brittle nails. Discuss any of these side effects with your doctor, especially if they are persistent or get worse.

Side effects from chemotherapy aren't insignificant, but they need not put your life on hold. Chemotherapy has improved to the point where a majority of working women—60 percent according to one survey—continue working during the course of their treatments. And if you just don't feel up to staying on the job, or you'd rather work part-time on a flexible schedule, discuss your options with your employer.

Hormone-Blocking Therapy

Some types of breast cancer are "fed" by the female hormones—estrogen, progesterone, or both. Hormone-blocking drugs can literally starve these cancers of their needed nutrients. They do this in one of two ways—by interfering with the body's production of estrogen, or by attaching to the hormone receptors of cancer cells. If the drug reaches the receptor first, there's no room for the hormone to attach. With no hormones to feed it, the cancer cell dies.

Hormone-blocking therapy is prescribed when blood tests show that hormone receptors are present, regardless of tumor size or lymph node involvement. One of the advantages of hormone-blocking therapy is that the drugs act against cancer cells without harming normal cells, making these drugs easier to tolerate than chemotherapy drugs.

Hormone-dependent tumor cells have *estrogen receptors* or *progesterone receptors*. Estrogen receptors and methods of blocking estrogen are better understood than progesterone receptors. Even so, women whose tumors have receptors for progesterone but not estrogen appear to benefit from estrogen-blocking therapies.

Hormone-blocking therapy improves a woman's prognosis by reducing the possibility of the same cancer recurring or a new cancer developing. With regular follow-up, the benefits of hormone-blocking therapy are likely to continue at least fifteen years after the five-year treatment period.

Tamoxifen

The drug most commonly used in hormone-blocking therapy is *tamoxifen* (Nolvadex), which belongs to a category of drugs called *selective estrogen receptor modulators (SERMs)*. These drugs block the effects of estrogen in breast tissue in premenopausal women. The first SERM to be developed, tamoxifen was approved for breast cancer treatment by the Food and Drug Administration in 1978 and remains the only FDA-approved drug for breast cancer prevention. To understand how tamoxifen works, it helps to think of a lock and key. The hormone receptors represent the "lock," and estrogen is the "key" that activates the cancer cells. Tamoxifen fits into the lock but, in effect, doesn't turn the lock; it just gets in the way of the key—the estrogen.

Though tamoxifen has been studied and used since the 1970s, first as a breast cancer treatment and more recently to prevent breast cancer, its precise mechanism isn't well understood. There is evidence that tamoxifen actually becomes incorporated into the cell and directly prevents the next cycle of cell division. The result is not just a temporary block but actual cell death.

To destroy as many cancer cells as possible, tamoxifen is given over a five-to-ten-year period, in a daily dose of 20 milligrams. Tamoxifen therapy usually begins within four weeks after surgery or chemotherapy, or immediately after radiation therapy has ended. Interestingly, while tamoxifen acts against estrogen in cancer cells, it acts very much like estrogen in preserving bone tissue, perhaps offering protection against osteoporosis.

Your doctor will give you a list of drugs to avoid while you're taking tamoxifen. Several drugs, ranging from certain antidepressants to anti-allergy medications, can affect the effectiveness of tamoxifen.

Other Hormone-Blocking Drugs

Other SERMs have been developed and continue to emerge as scientists attempt to replicate the benefits of tamoxifen without the side effects. *Raloxifene* (Evista), which is a drug approved for osteoporosis prevention, has been shown by studies to be as effective as tamoxifen in preventing breast cancer in high-risk postmenopausal women. Raloxifene carries a very slight risk of strokes that, although extremely rare, are more likely to be fatal.

Goserelin (Zoladex) is probably better known as a prostate-cancer drug. Just as it suppresses testosterone production in men, it suppresses estrogen production in premenopausal women, bringing on temporary menopause, with menopausal symptoms being the only side effects.

Aromatase inhibitors—*anastrozole* (Arimidex), *letrozole* (Femara), and *exemestane* (Aromasin)—block estrogen production in postmenopausal women by inhibiting the enzyme aromatase. Effective only in postmenopausal women, this enzyme converts other hormones to estrogen and is the body's principal source of estrogen after menopause. Arimidex is used either as a first hormone-blocking treatment or

> *Chemotherapy was relatively easy for me, and my family was considerate of my lack of energy. I bought a wig the same color as my hair and, for the most part, continued on with my life.*
> —*Carolyn, 65*

when other drugs, such as tamoxifen, have not fully halted the disease. Its side effects can include fatigue, hot flashes, nausea, back pain, bone pain, decreased bone density, some hair loss, and blood clots. Femara and Aromasin, also effective against tumors that resist tamoxifen, have milder side effects.

Side Effects of Hormone-Blocking Drugs

Your doctor will give you a list of possible side effects of hormone-blocking drugs; they include vaginal dryness, fatigue, depression, hot flashes, weight gain, insomnia, and memory loss.

Tamoxifen has been linked to a slightly higher risk of uterine cancer. You should not take tamoxifen if you have a history of blood clots. Years ago, when tamoxifen was prescribed in much higher doses, women taking the drug occasionally suffered eye damage. This side effect is extremely rare with today's lower doses, but you should still have regular eye exams while you are on tamoxifen.

Targeted Therapy

The term *targeted therapy* refers to the use of bioengineered drugs that interfere with cancer-causing mechanisms at the molecular level. Some targeted-therapy drugs represent truly astonishing accomplishments in genetic engineering. Side effects are typically mild because healthy cells aren't damaged.

Targeted-Therapy Drugs

The best-known drug used in targeted breast cancer therapy is *trastuzumab* (Herceptin). Approved by the FDA in 2006, Herceptin works on the surface of the cancer cell by blocking the chemical signals that can stimulate uncontrolled growth. However, the drug is recommended only for those women whose breast cancer tumors are HER2/neu-positive.

Herceptin is neither a hormonal therapy drug nor a chemotherapy drug. Rather, it is a *monoclonal antibody*—biologically engineered to act against the HER2/neu protein expressed by the HER2 gene. As described in chapter 2, HER2/neu "overexpression" is a factor in 20 to 30 percent of breast cancers, occurring when women have more than the normal pair of HER2 genes. These types of tumors tend to grow and spread more quickly than tumors that are not HER2/neu-positive.

Herceptin is given intravenously in a doctor's office. Infusions will usually last from thirty to ninety minutes, depending on your dosage, the frequency of your infusions, and how well you tolerate the infusions. The drug is added to a chemotherapy regimen and continues after the chemotherapy, for a total of one year.

Even though Herceptin may cause mild side effects, it does not cause hair loss or nausea, often associated with chemotherapy. In about 40 percent of women, the drug may cause flu-like symptoms such as fever, chills, nausea, or muscle aches; these symptoms usually diminish after the initial treatment. In rare cases, Herceptin may cause heart failure. In these cases, the drug can be stopped and the patient may regain full heart function with the help of heart-strengthening medications.

A newer drug called *lapatinib* (Tykerb) is also used in targeted breast cancer therapy. Tykerb, which blocks the HER1 and HER2 genes, is in the class of drugs called *tyrosine kinase inhibitors*. In simple terms, Tykerb blocks protein expression inside the cancer cell while Herceptin acts on protein on the cell's surface.

Is Systemic Therapy Right for You?

If you have not begun menopause, your doctor is more likely to prescribe chemotherapy than hormone-blocking therapy. For one thing, tumors in premenopausal women tend to lack hormone receptors—they are not dependent on hormones in order to grow. In addition, younger women tend to have faster-growing tumors than older women, and they have more years ahead of them in which cancer could recur. Chemotherapy can effectively reduce this long-term risk.

> *Breast cancer is like speed bumps in the road. You have rough days or rough procedures, but it gets better. You get over them.*
> —*Kristine, 51*

The reverse is true after menopause. Because their tumors are often slow-growing and hormone-dependent, postmenopausal women are more likely to receive hormone-blocking therapy.

Both therapies are given when conditions call for them. For example, a woman with a hormone-dependent cancer that has spread to the lymph nodes or is larger than one centimeter (less than half an inch) is likely to receive chemotherapy followed by hormone-blocking therapy, whether she is premenopausal or postmenopausal.

Research Continues

Scientists are eagerly pursuing targeted therapies using many different mechanisms to combat cancer. Some work by replacing missing or defective genes with "good" copies of the gene, sometimes using viruses as transportation. Other experimental targeted therapies use stem cells to deliver anticancer agents directly to tumor metastases, or vaccines to find and destroy cancer-promoting proteins.

Along with new drugs, refinements in genetic and molecular profiling of breast cancer make it possible to tailor treatment for the type of breast cancer a woman has. If you are seeking treatment, it is most helpful to find a medical oncologist who is aware of the latest news in cancer research so you can be assured of receiving the most current therapy. Treatments that were unimaginable twenty years ago are saving lives today.

8

If Cancer Recurs

If your breast cancer has responded well to therapy, you have every reason to celebrate—treatments have worked, you have survived, and your life can return to normal. However, if you are like most women, somewhere in the back of your mind you fear that the cancer will recur or that a new cancer will develop in your other breast. You may also worry that your breast cancer means your daughter, sister, mother, or granddaughter are at higher risk.

Some women first confront these kinds of fears when the initial shock of diagnosis wears off and surgery is over. Others don't begin worrying until they have finished radiation therapy or adjuvant therapy. When you stop making frequent visits to familiar doctors and nurses, you may feel strangely vulnerable. For example, you may feel a wave of anxiety with every small headache or bodily pain, certain that the cancer is back.

Fortunately, the intense anxieties subside with time. Most women begin relaxing a little after each checkup until two years, and then five, have finally passed. Although breast cancer has been known to recur as late as twenty-five years after the first diagnosis, it is most likely to reappear within the first five years, and especially the first two. After the ten-year mark, a woman's risk of recurrence is very small.

Risk of Recurrence

Keep in mind that 70 to 90 percent of the women diagnosed with early-stage breast cancer never have a recurrence after treatment. Well over half of the women who experience a recurrence live ten years or more after treatment for the recurrence. Here, again, early detection is key: The sooner a new tumor is discovered, the better the chances for recovery. Finally, there's a great deal you can do to keep your body strong and less vulnerable to recurrence.

In chapter 1, we discussed the general risks linked to primary breast cancer—the various environmental, hereditary, and behavioral factors thought to play a role in the development of this disease. To understand your risk of recurrence, consider these factors as well as the ones associated with your particular kind of breast cancer.

The same cancer characteristics that were used to guide your treatments will also help to estimate your risk of recurrence. These characteristics include:

- tumor size
- lymph node involvement
- presence or absence of hormone receptors
- rate of cancer-cell division (Poorly differentiated cells divide rapidly, well-differentiated cells divide less often.)
- presence of micrometastases
- HER2/neu overexpression
- BRCA1 or BRCA2 gene mutation
- Ki-67 and p53 tumor markers

Breast cancer can reappear at the site of the original tumor as a *local recurrence* or in another part of the body as a *distant recurrence,* or *metastasis.* Though it can spread to many different locations, the most common breast cancer metastases affect the lymph nodes, liver, lungs, and bones. After the lymph nodes, the bones are the most likely site for metastasis, apparently offering breast cancer cells a hospitable tissue and blood supply where they can multiply and thrive.

Ask your doctor about your specific risk of recurrence, realizing that, no matter how scientifically your risk factors and cancer characteristics are combined and analyzed, the outlook is only an indication, not a prediction. Cancer, by definition, is unpredictable, and most kinds of cancer cells have both "good" and "bad" traits, so it's impossible to be certain how a cancer

Preventing Cancer Recurrence

- Engage in three or more hours of moderate exercise each week.
- Eat a balanced, healthful diet.
- Control weight.
- Avoid alcohol.
- Control blood sugar, if diabetic.

will behave. Living each day with hope and a positive attitude can go a long way toward redeeming a less-than-positive prognosis.

One of the best strategies for long-term survival is to pay close attention to your body—using common sense, of course, so that you're not in a continual fret. Using the information in this book and other sources, you've learned the signs and symptoms of breast cancer. Now, become equally familiar with the warning signs of breast cancer recurrence. The better you understand the genuine warning signs, the more relaxed you'll probably be about unrelated symptoms.

Let your doctor know at once if you experience:

- bone pain
- headaches
- muscle weakness or numbness
- shortness of breath
- persistent cough
- weight loss or lack of appetite

Risk of a New Cancer

It is only fair to think that if you have had breast cancer once, you should not have to worry about it twice. But cancer is never fair, and sometimes a new primary cancer does develop, in a breast treated with lumpectomy, in the untreated breast, or, less commonly, in a small amount of breast tissue left behind after mastectomy. Fortunately, the risk of a second breast cancer remains small—about 0.5 to 1 percent per year after your first diagnosis. If you have had a very aggressive cancer, you may be more likely to develop breast cancer again.

There are some women who have an inherited tendency to develop a series of primary cancers. Those who have this unusual condition might recover from breast cancer only to face other cancers in other parts of the body. For information, talk with your doctor, or call the Hereditary Cancer Center (*see* the Resource section at the back of the book).

Follow-Up Care and Prevention

Physicians today have several strategies for reducing your risk of further cancer, and new strategies are being studied all the time. It is vitally important to continue getting the care you need, after your successful cancer treatment, to help catch any recurrence at its earliest stage. The danger of random, microscopic cancer cells remains, and if such cells find the right place to grow, they can form a new tumor.

Your follow-up care will be more frequent and comprehensive during the first year or so after your surgery. Depending on the treatment you received, you'll visit your cancer surgeon, radiation oncologist, medical oncologist, and plastic surgeon (if you have had reconstruction). Your primary physician, the one who has coordinated your care throughout your treatment, will probably be involved in your follow-up care as well. He or she should be in touch with all the members of your medical team throughout the follow-up period, and you'll probably see this doctor every six months or so for a complete physical examination. Your primary physician or other doctors may also order diagnostic tests as part of your follow-up care.

> *I always wonder if the cancer will return. I don't always talk about it, but the scare is there at times. One day at a time...that's how you live with cancer.*
>
> *—Liz, 42*

Blood Tests

After you have had systemic therapy, you'll probably have monthly blood tests until your blood counts stabilize. Your doctor might also use blood tests that look for *tumor markers,* abnormally high amounts of substances, such as certain kinds of proteins, that might indicate when a tumor is present. The tests are not sensitive enough to find a recurrence at its earliest stages, since a tumor must be large enough to release detectable amounts of the marker substances. Results sometimes include false negatives. Thus, the most appropriate use of these tests is in following a known recurrence to gauge its response to therapy.

Other blood tests look for elevated levels of enzymes that sometimes indicate the presence of cancer in the liver or bone. If test results suggest a problem with the liver, you may have a PET/CT scan to investigate further. If tests show that bone cancer could be present, or if you experience bone pain, your doctor will order a bone scan.

(Note: for women with early-stage breast cancers, routine scans are not recommended.)

Scans

The first step in a *bone scan* is injection of a harmless radioactive liquid into the bloodstream. After a few hours, the radioactive particles are taken up by the bones, where they concentrate in areas of increased blood circulation that could indicate cancer. Such areas, called "hot spots," are detected by a machine that scans your body from above while you are lying on a table. Hot spots can appear for many reasons— injury, arthritis, or other problems besides rapidly dividing cancer cells—and the machine cannot distinguish the cause. Therefore, if a bone scan finds an area of increased circulation, it will be followed up by an X-ray, PET/CT scan, or MRI, which can show more clearly what is going on at that site.

PET/CT Scan. This scan combines the PET scan with a CT scan, each test providing different information. The PET scan shows areas of increased metabolic activity while the CT scan shows physical detail. Equipment is now available that performs both scans at the same time; however, frequently the scans are done separately and their results are compiled into one report.

A *Computerized Tomography (CT)* uses radiation to display cross sections of the body, which can reveal cancers deep within the body or brain. During the scan, you'll need to lie very still while the CT machine takes X-ray pictures from many different angles. A computer assembles these slices of images into a detailed picture of the scanned area. In a spiral or helical CT scan, the X-ray beam rotates around you in a spiral. It is faster than a standard CT scan and may find smaller tumors.

Magnetic Resonance Imaging (MRI). An MRI uses magnets instead of X-rays to take many pictures from a variety of angles. The MRI can find soft-tissue abnormalities that other tests may overlook.

Chest X-Rays

Breast cancer survivors may be advised to have a chest X-ray if they experience shortness of breath or develop a persistent cough.

Breast Self-Examination and Mammography

Of course, self-examination and mammograms remain critical after cancer treatment. If you have had a lumpectomy, you should examine both breasts and the entire breast area, as outlined in chapter 2. If you have had a mastectomy, you should examine your untreated breast, the surgical site, and the surrounding area, paying attention to your incision and chest wall for thickness, lumps, or rigidity. Report any suspicious changes to your doctor immediately.

Most experts recommend a mammogram about six months after treatment. If you have had a lumpectomy, a mammogram of the surgically treated breast will serve as a new baseline. The other breast will look about the same on the new image as on earlier ones. If you have had a mastectomy, a physical examination of your incision, armpit, breast area, and the area above your collarbone

> *I chose a double mastectomy because I didn't want to have to worry about recurrence. I am glad I made the decision.*
>
> —*Billie, 48*

will be sufficient—but, of course, you should have routine mammograms done on your opposite breast. Most physicians recommend mammograms every six months for the first year or two after cancer treatment, and then annually after that.

Tamoxifen

If your original tumor tested positive for hormone receptors, you have probably begun a five-year course of hormone-blocking therapy, most likely with tamoxifen, which kills cancer cells by keeping them from dividing. Tamoxifen has not only been shown to prevent primary breast cancer in some high-risk women but also to keep it from recurring in women who have already had breast cancer. The drug also shrinks existing tumors and is used against breast cancer metastases. Like all anti-cancer drugs, it has risks and side effects as well as benefits, so you should ask your doctor to discuss these with you.

Pamidronate (Aredia)

A class of drugs called *bisphosphonates* disrupt the normal cycles in which bone breaks down and regenerates to keep the skeletal system healthy. *Pamidronate* (Aredia) is the most commonly prescribed bisphosphonate for this use. If your doctor thinks it would be beneficial in your case, you'll probably receive an injection of pamidronate every few weeks.

Treatment for Recurrence

The return of breast cancer to the original site or elsewhere in the body is called a *recurrence*. (If the reappearance of cancer actually represents cancer cells from the original tumor that weren't removed during treatment, then it's technically not a recurrence, though the remainder of this chapter will use the word "recurrence" to refer to newly active breast cancer from whatever cause.)

Local Recurrence

Cancer that reappears after lumpectomy, at the site of the original tumor, is one form of local recurrence. Radiation isn't an option for treating the cancer, since you will have had radiation after your lumpectomy, and repeated radiation would cause too much tissue damage. Your doctor will probably want to perform a mastectomy as the best way of removing all the cancer.

Local recurrence after mastectomy can appear in the surgical scar, in the skin or fat where the breast was, in the muscle or bone of the chest wall, or in a remnant of breast tissue left behind after the surgery. Surgery is the first line of treatment, to remove the cancer and any affected tissue, muscle, or bone. If you didn't have radiation to the site after your mastectomy, radiation can now be used on the entire breast area to eradicate any microscopic traces of the cancer.

Most cases of local recurrence are treated locally, with surgery and in some cases radiation. If the original tumor tested positive for hormone receptors, the woman will already be on a five-year regimen of tamoxifen or another hormone blocker. But if there is a chance that the local recurrence signals a wider metastasis, chemotherapy will be prescribed as well. For example, if the recurrence is in the mastectomy scar, the cancer has probably traveled there through the bloodstream and lymph nodes. The danger, of course, is that it has traveled elsewhere in the body as well. In this case, chemotherapy may halt any microscopic spread of the disease.

New chemotherapy drugs, in new combinations and dosages, are being tested and introduced all the time. Some of these are especially promising against recurrent cancer. The more your doctor stays informed about such developments, and aware of the conditions under which each drug or combination is most useful, the better he or she will be able to fine-tune your treatment and maximize its results.

You have to be an advocate for your own health. If you notice a change in your breast or a change in how you are feeling, get checked. We'd much rather have a false alarm than miss some- thing important.

—Stephen, medical oncologist

Metastasis, or Distant Recurrence

When breast cancer has spread to another part of the body, treatment must be as aggressive as possible, while keeping side effects tolerable. The same therapies are available for metastases as for a primary cancer—surgery, radiation (in areas not previously irradiated), and systemic therapies—though they may be used differently, and in different combinations or sequences, than with a primary cancer. Radiation is sometimes successful both in relieving the pain of metastases and in destroying the new tumor. In other cases, if a new tumor is localized and readily accessible to surgery, the recurrent cancer can be removed. Adjuvant therapies are used to decrease the incidence of inevitable metastatic disease.

Different systemic drugs may be used in different combinations for breast cancer metastases than for primary breast cancer. The focus among researchers is to develop new treatments that are at least as effective as ones currently in use, but with milder side effects and fewer risks.

Quality of Life

Whether your cancer recurs or you worry that it will, there are any number of things you can do to boost your confidence, protect your well-being, and feel in control over important aspects of your life. Many breast cancer survivors suggest living one day at a time, paying attention to the things that matter most—eating well, exercising, meditating, pursuing a spiritual search, finding creative expression, nurturing the relationships that sustain you—doing the things that fuel your energy and give you the greatest satisfaction. Try to reestablish routines and challenges that were interrupted by your illness. Add new ones, ways of reaching out and enriching your life.

When my cancer recurred, I was really angry. I told my sister, 'I can't do it.' But she convinced me that I did it once and I could do it again.
—Jean, 48

As mentioned in chapter 3, a support group can offer priceless help and new friendships. Consider working with organizations that promote breast cancer awareness and research. You might work with survivors like yourself or with women just recently diagnosed, who need to see what you represent—life going on. Activism has been responsible for many strides against breast cancer in recent years. You could make a difference by battling this disease on a new front, in small or energetic ways. There is always something you can do. Your life remains your own.

In Good Company
(An inner dialogue)

"What do you mean, it was cancer?"
(I am too busy for that.)

"Yes, I'll be there in the morning"
(I don't mind losing a breast.)

"Please turn the morphine pump higher"
(Oh my God, this really hurts.)

"Your chemo will last only six months"
(Oh, well, a baby takes nine.)

"Is that a wig? You look stunning!"
(Surely he's flattering me.)

"Welcome: Breast Cancer Support Group"
(I am in good company.)

—*Suzanne W. Braddock, M.D.*

Resources

American Society of Breast Surgeons
5950 Symphony Woods Road, Suite 212
Columbia, MD 21044
Phone: (410) 992-5470 or Toll free: (877) 992-5470
www.breastsurgeons.org
The American Society of Breast Surgeons Foundation is a charitable organization founded in 2005 dedicated to improving the standard of care for breast disease. It was established to support initiatives in the research and development of advanced breast disease treatments and technologies in order to improve the standards for superior patient care and education. They offer a state-of-the-art patient-access website for educational resources on breast disease awareness.

American Cancer Society (ACS)
15999 Clifton Road NE
Atlanta, GA 30329-4251
Phone: (800) ACS-2345 or (800) 227-2345
www.cancer.org
With more than two million volunteers and 3,400 local units, the ACS works to eliminate cancer as a major health problem through prevention, saving lives, and diminishing suffering through research, education, patient services, advocacy, and rehabilitation.

The ACS also sponsors the "Look Good. Feel Better," a free, nonmedical, brand-neutral, national public service program created to help individuals with cancer look good, improve their self-esteem, and manage their treatment and recovery with greater confidence. Visit www.lookgoodfeelbetter.org.

The American Cancer Society also sponsors the Hope Lodge in many cities; each Hope Lodge offers cancer patients and their families a free, temporary place to stay when their best hope for effective treatment may be in another city. For more information, visit www.cancer.org/treatment/supportprogramsservices/hopelodge/index.

Food and Drug Administration (FDA)
10903 New Hampshire Avenue
Silver Spring, MD 20993
(888) INFO-FDA or (888) 463-6332
www.fda.gov

The Food and Drug Administration is an federal agency of the United States Department of Health and Human Services and is responsible for protecting and promoting public health through the regulation and supervision of food safety, tobacco products, dietary supplements, prescription and over-the-counter pharmaceutical drugs, vaccines, biopharmaceuticals, and other products.

Hereditary Cancer Center (HCC)
Creighton University
Department of Preventative Medicine
2500 California Plaza
Omaha, NE 68178
Phone: (402) 280-2942
Fax: (402) 280-1734
http://medschool.creighton.edu/medicine/centers/hcc/index.php

The Hereditary Cancer Center (HCC) at Creighton University was established in 1984 in Omaha, Nebraska. The primary objective of the HCC is to conduct comprehensive research projects dealing with all types of cancer and is devoted to cancer prevention by identifying hereditary cancer syndromes. HCC conducts surveillance and management programs to oversee the natural history of these hereditary disorders.

National Cancer Institute (NCI)
National Institutes of Health
Bethesda, MD 20892-2580
Phone: (301) 496-4000
(800) 4-CANCER or (800) 422-6237
www.cancernet.nci.nih.gov

The NCI website offers recent cancer information from the National Cancer Institute, a component of the National Institutes of Health. Comprised of twenty-five separate institutes and centers, the NIH is one of eight health agencies in the U.S. Department of Health and Human Services.

National Coalition for Cancer Survivorship (NCCS)
1010 Wayne Avenue, Suite 315
Silver Spring, MD 20910-5600
Phone: (877) NCCS-YES
Fax: (301) 565-9670
www.canceradvocacy.org

Founded in 1986 by and for people with cancer and those who care for them, the National Coalition for Cancer Survivorship is a patient-led advocacy organization working on the behalf of people with all types of cancer and their families. Their mission is to ensure quality cancer care for all Americans by leading and strengthening the survivorship movement, empowering cancer survivors, and advocating for policy issues that affect cancer survivors' quality of life.

National Lymphedema Network, Inc.
225 Bush Street, Suite 357
San Francisco, CA 94104
Hotline: (800) 541-3259
Phone: (415) 908-3681
www.lymphnet.org

The Mission of the NLN is to create awareness of lymphedema through education and to promote and support the availability of quality medical treatment for all individuals at risk for or affected by lymphedema. Their website offers community groups and discussions, research and article archives, and support for finding treatment of lymphedema.

U.S. National Library of Medicine
8600 Rockville Pike
Bethesda, MD 20894
www.nlm.nih.gov/medlineplus
www.ncbi.nlm.nih.gov/pubmedhealth/

These two websites, MedlinePlus and PubMed Health, bring together authoritative information from the National Library of Medicine (NLM), the National Institutes of Health (NIH), and other government agencies and health-related organizations. Both sites provide easy access to medical journal articles and also have extensive information about drugs, an illustrated medical encyclopedia, interactive patient tutorials, and the latest health news.

Glossary

A

accelerated partial breast radiation: is radiation therapy delivered to only part of the breast over a period of days.

adjuvant therapy: anticancer drugs used in chemotherapy, hormone-blocking therapy, and targeted therapy, after surgery and/or radiation, to prevent recurrence or metastasis.

alkylators: a class of chemotherapy drugs that inhibit cell division and growth.

anastrozole (Arimidex): a drug used in hormone-blocking therapy.

anatomical implant: a breast implant that is fuller at the bottom than at the top; also called a teardrop, contoured, or shaped implant.

antimicrotubules: chemotherapy drugs that directly kill cancer cells with minimal damage to normal cells.

antineoplastics: chemotherapy drugs.

antitumor antibiotics: chemotherapy drugs.

areola: the darker-colored skin surrounding the nipple.

aromatase: an enzyme that converts other hormones to estrogen; it is the principal source of estrogen after menopause.

aromatase inhibitors: drugs that block estrogen production by inhibiting the hormone aromatase.

aspiration: a procedure in which a hollow needle withdraws fluid from a breast mass or other part of the body.

asymmetrical: having opposite sides or parts that do not precisely match, as when one breast is larger or smaller than the other.

axilla: armpit.

axillary dissection: surgical removal of lymph nodes in the armpit area.

B

baseline: a condition against which later changes are compared, as in a *baseline* mammogram, usually taken before age forty.

benign: not cancerous.

bilateral: having two sides; affecting two sides equally, as in a *bilateral* mastectomy.

biopsy: a diagnostic procedure that removes tissue for microscopic analysis.

bisphosphonates: a class of drugs that disrupt the normal cycle in which bone breaks down and regenerates.

bone marrow: soft cell tissue in the bone center, where red blood cells, white blood cells, and platelets are manufactured.

bone-marrow aspiration: the withdrawal of bone marrow to be analyzed for the presence of free-floating cancer cells.

bone scan: a diagnostic test that detects areas of increased blood circulation in the bone.

boost treatments: tightly focused, additional doses of radiation, usually given for a week or two after standard radiation treatments have ended.

brachytherapy: radiation treatment delivered to a precise location by a device implanted inside the body.

BRCA1, BRCA2: genes, which, when mutated, are associated with hereditary breast cancer.

breast implant: a soft pouch, filled with saline or silicone, that is surgically implanted beneath the skin and muscle of the chest wall to form a reconstructed breast after mastectomy.

breast reconstruction: any surgical method used to create a new breast after mastectomy. The new breast will not produce milk and will not have sensation but will look like a normal breast.

breast self-examination (BSE): a monthly routine in which a woman follows several steps to detect any changes or suspicious lumps in her breasts.

bulb: the smallest component in the milk-producing system of lobes in the breast.

C

cancer: a general term for diseases characterized by uncontrolled growth of abnormal cells that can invade and destroy healthy tissue. Also called *malignancy*.

capsular contracture: a complication following implant reconstruction in which scar tissue around the implant begins to contract and squeeze the implant.

carcinogenic: cancer-causing.

carcinoma: the most common type of cancer, affecting skin, glands, or the lining of organs.

catheter: a tube-shaped medical device inserted into the body to keep a passage open or to facilitate the injection or withdrawal of fluids.

cell: the smallest structural unit of living tissue that can survive and reproduce on its own.

cell cycle: all cell activity from one cell division to the next.

chemotherapy: the administration of anticancer drugs that directly kill cancer cells or disrupt their ability to grow and reproduce.

clinical trial: a research project that tests drugs or other treatments on human subjects.

core biopsy: a diagnostic test in which a hollow needle removes small samples of tissue for laboratory analysis.

CT (computerized tomography) scan: a computer-aided method of creating three-dimensional images of organs and structures inside the body.

cyclophosphamide: an alkylator.

cytologist: a specialist who analyzes cells and diagnoses disease from cell abnormalities.

cytotoxic: toxic to cells; capable of destroying cells.

cyst: a benign, fluid-filled lump.

D

DCIS (ductal carcinoma *in situ*): a precancerous condition in which abnormal cells have been found in the milk ducts of the breast but have not broken through the duct walls.

density: compact, thick.

DES (diethylstilbestrol): a synthetic estrogen that was once prescribed to prevent complications in pregnancy; it is no longer used because it increases the risk of breast cancer.

diagnosis: the process of identifying a disease from its symptoms and from tests such as X-rays or biopsies; in breast cancer, determining the nature of a lump or any other change in the breast.

diagnostic mammogram: not a routine mammogram, but one ordered to investigate a lump found during BSE or a clinical examination.

DIEA flap (deep inferior epigastric artery): a section of skin and fat moved up from the lower abdomen to the chest area and used for breast reconstruction after mastectomy.

diffuse: not localized in a single area.

digital mammography: a process in which the images produced on a mammogram machine are converted to computer code and then displayed in much finer detail than film can capture.

distant recurrence: a reappearance of cancer at a site other than the site of the original tumor.

DNA (deoxyribonucleic acid): the material that carries the genetic code, and establishes hereditary patterns, including inherited risks for certain diseases.

DNA repair enzyme inhibitors: chemotherapy drugs.

duct: a narrow tube that carries milk from the lobes of the breast to the nipple.

ductal carcinoma: cancer that arises in the milk ducts.

ductal lavage: a diagnostic test in which a saline solution is introduced into the breast ducts and then withdrawn so that cells from the ducts can be analyzed for abnormalities.

E

early detection: discovery of a cancer while it is still small—no more than two centimeters (less than an inch) in diameter—and before it has spread to lymph nodes near the breast.

enzyme: a complex protein that supports or initiates certain chemical reactions in the body.

epidermal growth factor receptor (EGRF): This cell-surface protein is a receptor for members of the epidermal growth factor family.

erythropoietin: a drug that stimulates the production of red blood cells.

estrogen: a female sex hormone produced by the ovaries, adrenal glands, placenta, and fatty tissues.

estrogen receptor: a location on a tumor at which estrogen molecules can attach; the presence of estrogen receptors means a tumor depends on estrogen to grow.

excisional biopsy: a surgical biopsy used for small tumors and capable of removing them completely.

exemestane (Aromasin): a drug used in hormone-blocking therapy; it blocks estrogen production in postmenopausal women by inhibiting the enzyme aromatase.

expander: a soft, empty pouch placed behind the chest muscle and gradually filled with saline over a period of months to stretch the skin before a breast implant is put in place.

external beam brachytherapy: a treatment that delivers radiation to a tumor area but requires no catheters or balloons.

external boost treatment: external beam radiation therapy delivered to a smaller area after a course of standard radiation therapy.

external radiation: radiation delivered from outside the body.

extrusion: the act of being forced through an opening, such as when an implant extrudes due to skin erosion.

F

false positive: a test that erroneously shows a positive result.

fibrocystic changes: a common condition in which the breasts develop benign, normal cysts that are sometimes mistaken for suspicious lumps. Often called fibrocystic disease, this condition is not actually an illness.

filgrastim: a drug that stimulates the production of red blood cells.

fine-needle aspiration (FNA): a kind of biopsy in which fluid is withdrawn (aspirated) using a fine, hollow needle. In the case of breast cancer, the fluid is aspirated from a tumor, and the cells within the fluid are examined for evidence of cancer.

G

genetic: having to do with the genes and hereditary characteristics.

gluteal flap: a wedge of skin, muscle, and fat taken from the buttocks to be used in breast reconstruction.

goserelin: a drug that suppresses estrogen production in premenopausal women.

graft: to surgically implant living tissue.

guided imagery: any of a number of techniques used to visualize images or imagine sensations in an effort to trigger a desired physical effect.

H

hematoma: a mass of blood that collects in tissue or organs; breasts may be susceptible to hematomas after surgery.

Herceptin: a drug developed for women with HER2-positive breast cancer.

hereditary: genetically passed on by a parent or parents to offspring; the risk for some cancers is hereditary.

HER2/neu: a gene that helps control how cells grow, divide, and repair themselves, important in the control of abnormal or defective cells that could become cancerous.

hormone: a substance secreted by glands and circulated in the bloodstream to other parts of the body, where it exerts specific effects on cell activity.

hormone-blocking therapy: the use of drugs that block or disrupt the body's production of hormones in cases where a tumor depends on those hormones to grow.

hormone receptors: a location on a tumor at which either estrogen or progesterone molecules can attach; the presence of hormone receptors means a tumor depends on hormones to grow.

hyperplasia: uncontrolled, abnormally fast growth of cells.

hypofractionated radiation therapy: an accelerated course of radiation therapy, with higher doses given over the period of a few days.

I

image-guided biopsy: a technique in which computer images are used to guide a biopsy needle to a lump that cannot be felt but has shown up on a mammogram; also called a stereotactic biopsy.

immunohistochemical staining: a process in which living cells and tissues can be analyzed.

incisional biopsy: an open biopsy in which a small piece of a tumor is removed for laboratory analysis.

industry-based trials: a type of clinical trial sponsored by pharmaceutical companies in compliance with FDA requirements.

inflammatory breast cancer: a particularly aggressive form of breast cancer usually treated with chemotherapy before surgery.

infusion: slow drip of medication directly into a vein.

inhibitors: an agent used to reduce or slow the activity of a substance.

in situ: a term meaning "in position" or "in its place"; a breast cancer that has not spread through the wall of the milk duct or lobe where it originated is called *in situ*.

internal boost treatment: radiation therapy delivered internally to a small area after a course or standard radiation therapy.

invasive: cancer that is capable of invading, or has invaded, breast tissue beyond the wall of the duct or lobe in which it has arisen.

K

Ki-67: a protein whose growth rate in cancer cells can be measured to help determine how fast a tumor is growing.

L

lactation: milk production in the breast.

lapatinib: a drug sold as Tykerb used as a targeted breast cancer therapy.

latissimus dorsi flap: a section of muscle, skin, and some fat taken from the latissimus dorsi muscle of the upper back and used to form a new breast after mastectomy.

LCIS (lobular carcinoma *in situ*): the presence of abnormal cells within a lobe or lobes of one or both breasts; the cells have not spread beyond the walls of any lobes. The presence of LCIS indicates a heightened risk for either invasive lobular or ductal cancer.

letrazole *(Femara)*: a drug used in hormone-blocking therapy; it blocks estrogen production in postmenopausal women by inhibiting the enzyme aromatase.

linear accelerator: the machine most commonly used to deliver radiation treatments.

lobe: one of fifteen to twenty rounded divisions in each breast; the part of the breast in which milk is produced.

lobular carcinoma: cancer that originates in the milk-producing lobules of the breast.

lobule: one of several small components of a lobe.

local cancer: cancer that is occurring only one part of the body.

local recurrence: reappearance of cancer at the site of the original tumor.

local treatment: treatment of cancer at the site of the tumor by surgery or radiation.

lumpectomy: breast cancer surgery that removes only the tumor and a surrounding margin of healthy tissue to be examined for cancer cells; also called a wide excision or partial mastectomy.

lymph, lymphatic fluid: a clear, yellowish fluid containing white blood cells that bathes body tissues and carries waste products away through lymph vessels.

lymphedema: a persistent swelling caused by excess fluid that may collect when the lymph nodes and vessels are removed. This condition can occur at any time after surgery, including years later.

lymph nodes: small masses of lymphatic tissue distributed along the lymph vessels and containing lymphocytes that filter waste products from lymphatic fluid.

lymph vessels: similar to blood vessels but with the purpose of circulating lymphatic fluid through the body and to the lymph nodes.

M

malignant: cancerous.

MammaPrint: molecular diagnostic test that is used to assess the risk that a breast tumor will spread to other parts of the body.

mammogram: an image of the breast created by mammography.

mammography: the use of X-rays to examine the breasts for tumors or microcalcifications.

Mammotome: a biopsy that uses suction and a large tube to withdraw breast tissue; also called vacuum-assisted biopsy.

margin: healthy tissue surrounding a tumor, removed at the same time as the tumor for laboratory analysis.

marker: a mechanism that identifies, characterizes, or predicts.

mastectomy: surgical removal of the breast.

mastitis: infection of the breast.

medical oncologist: a physician who specializes in systemic cancer treatments.

menopause: the permanent cessation of menstrual periods, usually in a woman's late forties to early fifties.

metachronous: occurring in a series.

metastasis: the spread of cancer from its original site to another part of the body or lymphatic system.

metastasizing: spreading to other parts of the body.

microcalcifications: tiny, grain-sized deposits of calcium in breast tissue, detectable by mammogram; when they appear in clusters, they are a sign of DCIS.

microcatheter: an extremely small tube used in ductal lavage.

micrometastasis: the early spread of cancer from the original tumor by means of random, microscopic cancer cells that have not yet formed a mass and are generally not detectable. (However, bone-marrow aspiration can detect micrometastases when the cancer has begun to spread to bone.)

microtubule: very small tubules within the cytoplasm of a cell.

microtubule inhibitors: a chemotherapy drug.

modified radical mastectomy: surgery that removes the entire breast and the axillary lymph nodes.

monoclonal antibody: an antibody derived from a single cell to act against a certain antigen.

MRI (magnetic resonance imaging): a diagnostic imaging test that uses a powerful magnet and radio waves to show differences in the number of blood vessels in various types of body tissue. Cancerous tissue tends to have more blood vessels than healthy tissue.

multifocal: having more than one location; a multifocal breast cancer is present simultaneously in more than one lobe or duct.

mutation: a change in a cell's DNA.

myocutaneous: comprising muscle, skin, and fat; a myocutaneous flap is taken from one part of the body to reconstruct another, such as a surgically removed breast.

N

negative biopsy: a biopsy in which no cancer cells are seen in the tissue or fluid removed.

neoadjuvant therapy: chemotherapy or hormone-blocking therapy given before surgery to shrink a tumor to operable size.

neoplasia: the process in which a tumor forms.

nipple: the portion of the breast that protrudes and through which milk is drawn.

nipple-areola: the nipple and surrounding shaded area.

node-negative: showing no evidence of cancer in the lymph nodes. A breast tumor is deemed node-negative when axillary dissection or sentinel node biopsy finds no cancer cells.

non-opioid: non-narcotic.

O

oncogene: a mutated gene associated with a heightened risk of cancer.

oncologist: a medical doctor who specializes in cancer treatment.

Oncotype DX: a diagnostic test that quantifies the likelihood of disease recurrence in women with early-stage breast cancer.

open biopsy: any surgical biopsy.

opioid: narcotic.

osteoporosis: a disease in which the bones become more porous and more susceptible to breakage as a person ages.

P

Pamidronate: one of a class of drugs called bisphosphonates, which have been shown in some studies to prevent the spread of breast cancer to bone or to treat the cancer effectively if it does spread.

pathologist: a medical specialist who analyzes biopsied tissue under a microscope and diagnoses disease from any abnormalities that are present.

pathology report: the pathologist's written record of the analysis of biopsied tissue.

peau d'orange: skin texture like that of an orange; a symptom of inflammatory breast cancer.

pectoralis minor: a small, strap-like muscle running from the outer edge of the collarbone to the top of the breast, sometimes removed during axillary dissection.

pegfilgrastim: a drug given in conjunction with chemotherapy to lessen its toxic effects.

PET (positron emission tomography scan): a diagnostic imaging test that reveals cell activity by detecting the different rates at which different cells consume sugar, or glucose. Cancer cells consume glucose more rapidly than normal cells.

p53 gene: a gene that normally acts as a tumor suppressor but when abnormal, may be associated with a high risk of breast cancer.

phantom breast: the sensation that a surgically removed breast is still present.

plant alkaloid: chemotherapy drugs.

plastic surgeon: a specialist in cosmetic and reconstructive surgery.

platelets: blood cells that aid clotting.

polygenic breast cancer: cancer that usually shows up in more than one member of an extended family.

port: a small, semipermanent opening that is surgically implanted just under the skin. It is attached to a tube leading directly to a large vein. A port may be used when repeated injections are necessary, since it eliminates the need to tap a new vein each time.

postmenopausal: after menopause.

preinvasive: malignant cells that are capable of becoming invasive but have yet to spread into surrounding tissues.

premenopausal: before menopause.

primary cancer: a first-occurring tumor.

progesterone: a female sex hormone produced by the ovaries.

progesterone receptor: a location on a tumor at which progesterone molecules can attach.

progestin: synthetic progesterone.

prognosis: the likely outcome of a disease; in the case of breast cancer, the statistical chance of long-term, disease-free survival.

prophylactic: preventive; a prophylactic mastectomy is performed when no cancer is present but the risk of breast cancer is high.

prosthesis: an external breast form worn by some women after mastectomy.

protocol: a document listing all steps, procedures, safety measures, and research methods to be used in a clinical trial.

Q

quadrant: any of the four segments into which a body part can be divided vertically and horizontally.

quadrantectomy: a partial mastectomy involving removal

of the quadrant of the breast in which the tumor is located.

quality-of-life trials: a type of clinical trial that focuses on issues such as pain management and chronic side effects.

R

radiation oncologist: a medical doctor who specializes in radiation therapy.

radiation pneumonitis: a short-term inflammation of lung tissue caused by exposure to radiation therapy.

radiation therapy: a local treatment in which a radioactive beam is used to kill cancer cells in the area of the tumor.

radical mastectomy: an invasive surgical procedure that removes the breast, the axillary lymph nodes, and the muscle of the chest wall; radical mastectomy is almost never used today.

radiologist: a medical doctor who specializes in the interpretation of X-ray images for diagnosis.

raloxifene: one of the class of drugs called SERMs, used in hormone-blocking therapy.

receptors: a cell or a group of cells to which the hormones estrogen and progesterone can attach themselves.

reconstructive surgery: the use of plastic surgery to model a new breast after mastectomy, using either breast implants or tissue from elsewhere in the body. The reconstructed breast looks like a normal breast but is not functional and does not have sensation.

recurrence: the reappearance of cancer after an initial course of treatment has ended; recurrence can be local or distant.

red blood cells: cells that carry oxygen, which gives the body fuel for energy.

retraction: a drawing-in or drawing-back; when the nipple or the skin of the breast retracts, it can be a sign of inflammatory breast cancer.

S

saline: a sterile, saltwater solution.

screening mammogram: a routine mammogram usually performed annually to check for indications of breast cancer.

sentinel node: the first lymph node to which lymphatic fluid drains from the area of a tumor; therefore, the first in which spreading cancer cells are likely to show up.

sentinel node biopsy: a procedure that removes a sample of tissue from the sentinel node for examination under a microscope. If the sentinel node is free of cancer, the other nodes do not need to be removed and examined, and surgery is minimized.

sentinel node mapping: locating the sentinel node.

SERM (selective estrogen receptor modulator): one of a category of drugs that block either hormone production in the body or the hormone receptors on tumors, thus depriving certain cancers of the hormones they need for growth.

side effect: an undesirable effect of surgery, chemotherapy, radiation, or other treatment; some side effects include pain, nausea, skin changes, hair loss, or fatigue.

silicone: a synthetic material used to encase and fill some breast implants.

simple bilateral mastectomy: the surgical removal of all breast tissue from both breasts with no removal of lymph nodes; also called total bilateral mastectomy.

simple mastectomy: the surgical removal of all breast tissue but no lymph nodes; also called total mastectomy.

spiculated: star-shaped; a spiculated mass on a mammogram that should be biopsied for cancer cells.

spiral CT scan: a CT scan in which the X-ray beam rotates around you in a spiral; also called helical CT scan.

sporadic breast cancer: breast cancer in a patient with no known family history of the disease.

stage: the grading system for the severity of a disease.

stage migration: when breast cancer is identified as being at a different stage in its development due to new breast cancer staging guidelines.

stem cell rescue: drugs given to stimulate the production of bone-marrow stem cells.

stem cell transplant: a procedure for regenerating bone marrow destroyed by high doses of chemotherapy drugs. Bone-marrow stem cells (cells capable of forming blood cells) are removed before chemotherapy and then reintroduced afterward to restore bone marrow and its production of blood cells.

stereotactic biopsy: a technique in which computer images are used to guide a biopsy needle to a lump that cannot be felt but has shown up on a mammogram; also called image-guided biopsy.

submuscular: the placement of a breast implant beneath the pectoral muscle.

surgical biopsy: using an incision for the removal of part or all of a lump or suspicious area to be examined by a pathologist; also called open biopsy.

symmetry shapers: products that can be placed in a bra to achieve a symmetrical appearance post-mastectomy; also called "balance shapers."

synchronous: occurring at the same time.

systemic treatment: a cancer treatment such as chemotherapy that travels throughout the body to destroy random, microscopic cancer cells that may have spread beyond the site of the original tumor.

T

tamoxifen: an estrogen-blocking drug used in treating and preventing breast cancer.

targeted therapy: administration of a drug created to target cancer cells.

taxane: one of several chemotherapy drugs that directly kill cancer cells with minimal damage to healthy cells.

temporary radiation implants: small catheters used to deliver radiation.

tissue expander: a temporary balloon-like device, made of elastic silicone rubber, used to stretch the skin in the breast area following mastectomy.

tissue expansion: a process in which a soft, empty pouch is placed behind the chest muscle and gradually filled with saline over a period of months; this stretches the skin to accommodate a breast implant.

tomosynthesis: an FDA-approved, digital screening test for breast cancer. Also referred to as 3-D mammography, it provides a clearer picture of breast tissues than a regular mammogram.

topoisomerase inhibitor: a chemotherapy drug.

total mastectomy: the surgical removal of all breast tissue but no lymph nodes; also called simple mastectomy.

toxic: poisonous.

TRAM flap: a section of muscle, skin, and fat moved up from the lower abdomen to the chest area and used for breast reconstruction after mastectomy.

transducer: a microphone-like device that's passed over the skin during an ultrasound test.

trastuzumab: Herceptin.

tumor: an abnormal growth of cells or tissue. Tumors can be benign (noncancerous) or malignant (cancerous).

Tykerb: brand name for the drug lapatinib, used in targeted breast cancer therapy. It interupts HER2/neu and EGFR pathways.

tyrosine kinase inhibitor: a drug used in targeted therapy.

U

ultrasonography: the use of high-frequency sound waves to generate images of internal organs or tumors. Ultrasonography can determine whether a suspicious lump is filled with fluid or is solid; if it is solid, it could be cancerous and should be tested further.

V

vascular: of or relating to blood vessels.

visualization: the formation of visual images.

W

white blood cells: cells that fight infection.

wide excision: removal of a breast tumor and surrounding margin of normal tissue; also called a lumpectomy.

Index

Index

Index

Index

About the Authors

Suzanne W. Braddock, M.D., has been a breast cancer survivor since 1992. She is a dermatologist in private practice in Omaha, Nebraska. Born and raised in New Jersey, Dr. Braddock received her medical training at the Medical College of Pennsylvania, Philadelphia, and at the University of Nebraska Medical School, Omaha. Dr. Braddock is the author of several scientific publications. She has a daughter, Gail. For more information about Dr. Braddock, visit **www.braddockfinnegandermatology.com.**

Jane Kercher, M.D., F.A.C.S., is a general and oncological surgeon in Denver, Colorado. She received her medical training at the University of Utah Medical School, Salt Lake City, and at the University of Nebraska Medical School, Omaha. A native of Wyoming, Dr. Kercher now lives in Denver with her son, Matthew. For more information about Dr. Kercher, visit **www.SurgOne.com.**

John J. Edney, M.D. F.A.C.S., a plastic surgeon in private practice in Omaha, Nebraska, specializes in postmastectomy breast reconstruction and cosmetic surgery. Dr. Edney is the Chief of the Division of Plastic Surgery at the Nebraska Methodist Hospital. He is an assistant Clinical Professor of Surgery at the University of Nebraska Medical School, Omaha, and Creighton University School of Medicine. Dr. Edney and his wife, Pat, have three children—Christopher, Matthew, and Jennifer. Dr. Edney may be contacted through his website, **www.surgicalimages. com.**

Margaret Block, M.D., F.A.C.P., is a medical oncologist with Nebraska Cancer Specialists in Omaha, Nebraska. Board-certified in both internal medicine and medical oncology, Dr. Block treats many women with breast cancer. She is a native of New York City and attended Albany Medical College in Albany, New York; she received her medical oncology training at the University of Wisconsin in Madison, Wisconsin. Dr. Block is a member of the United States Oncology Breast Cancer Committee. She also serves on several local breast cancer boards. For more information, visit: **www.nebraskacancer.com**

Melanie Morrissey Clark has worked as a writer and editor for more than twenty years. She is also coauthor of *The Fertility Handbook—A Guide to Getting Pregnant* (Addicus Books, 2002). Ms. Clark is vice president of Clark Creative Group in Omaha. She holds a bachelor of science degree in journalism from the University of Nebraska. She lives in Omaha with her husband, Fred Clark, and their triplets, Cooper, Sophie, and Simon.

Consumer Health Titles from Addicus Books

Visit our online catalog at www.AddicusBooks.com

Understanding Parkinson's Disease, 2nd Edition $19.95

Understanding Peyronie's Disease. $16.95

Understanding Your Living Will $12.95

A Woman's Guide to Cosmetic Breast Surgery and Body Contouring $21.95

Your Complete Guide to Breast Augmentation & Body Contouring $21.95

Your Complete Guide to Breast Reduction and Breast Lifts $21.95

Your Complete Guide to Facial Rejuvenation. $21.95

Your Complete Guide to Nose Reshaping $21.95

To Order Books:
Visit us online at: www.AddicusBooks.com
Call toll free: (800) 888-4741